RELENTLESS

RELENTLESS

How a Leading
New York City Health System
Mobilized to Battle
the Greatest Health Crisis
of Our Era

Deborah Schupack

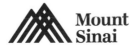
Mount
Sinai

This book may be purchased in bulk for educational purposes through the HFS Books website, https://www.hfsbooks.com/books/relentless-schupack/.

Library of Congress Cataloging-in Publication Data is available on file.

Cover design: Robert Matza
Book design: Priest + Grace

Print ISBN: 978-0-578-95838-5

Printed in the United States of America

To health care workers, in awe and with gratitude

CONTENTS

PART 3

THE URGENCY OF SCIENCE

PART 4

BUILDING THE FUTURE OF HEALTH CARE

AUTHOR'S NOTE

THERE ARE MANY CHALLENGES in committing words to a page about the largest pandemic in modern times while the world is still in the grips of the virus. COVID-19 and the battle against it followed no seasonal timetable, did not observe day or night, held no sacred boundaries. The ending to the story is far from certain. In fact, we don't even know how close to an ending we are. The recorded global death toll from COVID-19 stands today—on August 13, 2021—at more than 4.3 million, with the case count at 205.6 million, although the actual numbers are thought to be much, much higher. Variants, which happen over time with such a widespread virus, began changing the trajectory and pace of spread. Health care systems in many regions of the United States and the world were still (or again) overwhelmed with patients more than a year and a half after the first reports of the novel coronavirus in humans. Treatments for the most severe patients were still elusive, supplies still limited, and deaths still mounting. Societies and economies were still reopening and closing again with great turbulence.

The development of remarkably effective vaccines in record time changed the course of the virus for much of vaccinated society. Vaccinations for Mount Sinai health care workers began on December 15, 2020, and proceeded apace through 2021 for employees, patients, and community members, as well as for billions of people nationally and globally. The United States and the United Kingdom were among the limited number of countries that had enough vaccine supply to meet the demand of the general public, but much of the world struggled with access to vaccines. Even in places where plenty of vaccines were available, including the United States, many people elected to remain unvaccinated. Children under twelve were still not eligible for vaccination. Over the summer of 2021, the pandemic was characterized as a race between vaccines and variants.

This book delimits the still-unfolding story to that of the first pandemic year, 2020, zooming in on, in particular, the first devastating wave that hit New York City in March through May. These pages also explore the preparation beforehand, the science that began as soon as the virus's sequence was released in January (building on existing research projects and partnerships), and complex clinical, operational, and scientific activity that continued throughout 2020. The book cannot help but turn the corner into 2021, chronicling evolving scientific discoveries, clinical updates, and operational changes that bear reporting and shed light on lessons learned from this defining moment, trends and shifts begun or accelerated, and new directional commitments that might help the Mount Sinai Health System—and the greater health care universe—better weather the future shocks that are certainly coming our way.

FOREWORD

THIS IS A STORY OF COURAGE, resilience, and determination, a story about heroes—thousands of heroes—who bravely stepped forward to engage in a life-and-death battle against a lethal virus, the severe acute respiratory syndrome coronavirus 2 (SARS-CoV-2), and the infectious disease it causes, COVID-19, which has killed millions of people worldwide.

The Mount Sinai Hospital identified New York City's first case of COVID 19 on February 29, 2020. Within days, COVID-19 would hit the city with the force of a tsunami, and Mount Sinai Health System—a tightly knit network of eight hospitals, clinics, and the Icahn School of Medicine at Mount Sinai—would become ground zero for the first wave of the pandemic in the United States, an unprecedented medical emergency that brought New York to its knees.

From the doctors, nurses, and respiratory therapists fighting on the front lines to the research scientists who unraveled the mysteries of COVID-19 and the health system leaders who mobilized clinical and research armies, this is the complete account of how Mount Sinai rose to meet the challenge of COVID-19.

When it struck, COVID-19 was an unknown enemy. We did not know the origin of the virus or its precise mode of transmission. Most importantly, we did not know how to treat COVID-19.

We did know that SARS-CoV-2 was highly contagious and deadly. Even so, our team members did not hesitate to serve. In an all-hands-on-deck situation, they overcame fear with New York grit, launching into action to care for severely ill patients, help them breathe, clear their arteries, transport them, sanitize their rooms, comfort them, and serve as surrogate family because their loved ones could not be permitted to visit them in the hospital. Everyone helped however they could. Skilled surgeons carried oxygen tanks; engineers built dozens of negative-pressure rooms to contain the virus; medical students triaged patients; and administrators and board members hunted down essential personal protective equipment halfway around the globe.

Researchers, in constant collaboration with Mount Sinai clinicians, fought COVID-19 with science. In their laboratories, they worked tirelessly to understand the disease and determine how best to treat it, enabling the Health System to rapidly mount a strong counterattack.

Early in the pandemic, Mount Sinai scientists saw how COVID-19 attacks the endothelial cells lining the blood vessels, greatly increasing the likelihood of clots. This led to Mount Sinai's early decision to use anticoagulants for critically ill COVID-19 inpatients, which would save many lives and become a standard of care worldwide. Mount Sinai scientists quickly recognized that excessive inflammation in COVID-19 patients causes organ damage. So they created a rapid test to measure each patient's inflammatory response and guide treatment. They developed another test to measure not only the presence but also the precise level of COVID-19 antibodies in an individual, an assay that became the world's gold standard. They invented an inexpensive vaccine, in clinical trials in Vietnam, Thailand, Brazil, and Mexico as of this writing, which has the potential to protect low- and middle-income nations against the pandemic. These results, among others detailed in this book, demonstrate the critical importance of science to the advancement of medicine and its ability to save lives.

From scientists to sanitation workers, physicians to pharmacists, the employees of Mount Sinai Health System worked through exhaustion. They worked through fear. They did not stand down.

We are privileged to work alongside such committed and compassionate workers whose deeply embedded moral compass drives them to serve, to give it their all, especially at our hour of greatest need. In every sense of the word they are heroes.

Heroism, though, does not come without costs. For some, the cost was far too great. Tragically, more than 25 members of the Mount Sinai family fell to COVID-19. We mourn their loss and present this book as testimony to their brave sacrifice, which saved the lives of so many others.

The death of colleagues and patients was traumatic for our front-line health care workers. You will read of events that are forever etched in their memories. As courageous and resilient as they are, it is natural that some of them have experienced symptoms of post-traumatic stress disorder. This is why Mount Sinai established the Center for Stress, Resilience, and Personal Growth just two months after COVID-19 arrived in New York to help our employees put their experiences in perspective and fortify their resilience as they navigate through feelings of loss and anxiety.

Many of the stories you will read involve patients who are Black and Latinx. Their communities were disproportionately impacted by COVID-19, a fact that highlights long-standing health disparities in the United States. This is an issue that must be addressed. Mount Sinai's Institute for Health Equity Research is collaborating with policymakers, health care providers, and insurance companies to deliver actionable solutions that can improve health and access to care across the nation's demographic divide. We invite others to join us in this quest to resolve health inequities.

We hope this book will serve as a source of inspiration and learning for our colleagues in health care, at hospitals and clinics, medical schools and research institutions, regulatory bodies, and health care companies of all kinds. You are our partners in the continuing fight to defeat the global pandemic and advance science for the benefit of patients. Within this book are details of steps that were essential to Mount Sinai's response to the pandemic. Among them:

- **Mobilization.** By redeploying health care workers and reallocating resources we rapidly transformed an eight-hospital health system into a citywide emergency care center that could effectively manage a deluge of critically ill patients.
- **Improvisation.** We quickly redesigned patient rooms, trans-

formed buildings, and creatively reconfigured medical equipment to accommodate as many patients as necessary. Creative thinking became the order of the day as we reassessed established protocols.

- **Collaboration.** Mount Sinai's commitment to dynamic collaboration between biomedical researchers and clinicians, and across departments, proved to be more important than ever as physicians relied upon our latest laboratory insights to determine the course of treatment for patients.

- **Acceleration.** Under immense pressure, we rapidly accelerated our scientific analyses and their application to medical practice. Translational research benefited patients in a matter of days, rather than months or years.

Lastly, this story of Mount Sinai's response to COVID-19 provides insight to patients, their families, and all health care consumers, who are entitled to know of their providers' deep commitment to deliver the best in care and of the scientists who dedicate their lives to generating breakthroughs that improve medicine.

KENNETH L. DAVIS, MD
Chief Executive Officer
Mount Sinai Health System

DENNIS S. CHARNEY, MD
Anne and Joel Ehrenkranz Dean
Icahn School of Medicine at Mount Sinai
President for Academic Affairs
Mount Sinai Health System

MARGARET PASTUSZKO, MBA
President and Chief Operating Officer
Mount Sinai Health System

PART 1

A CLINICAL MISSION OF EPIC PROPORTIONS

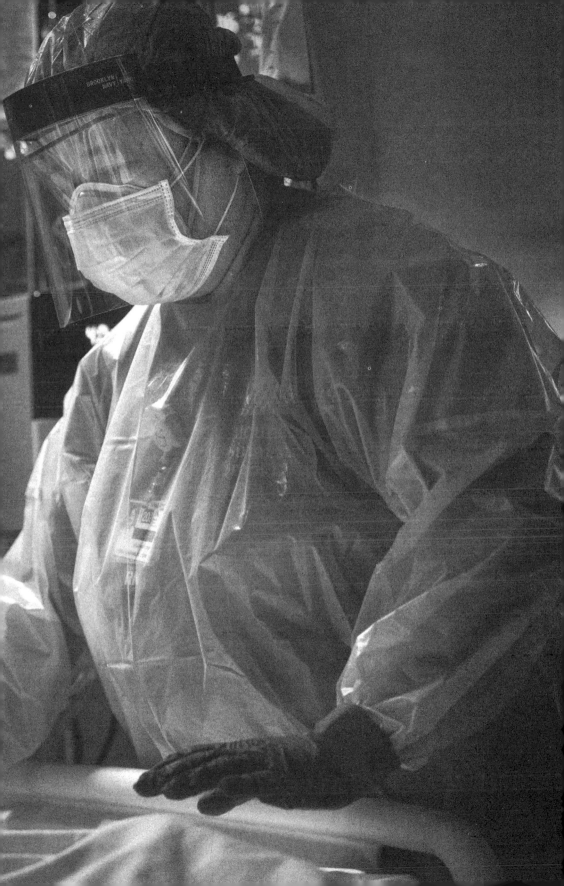

1 | COVID-19 SURFACES IN NEW YORK CITY

'I think this is it'

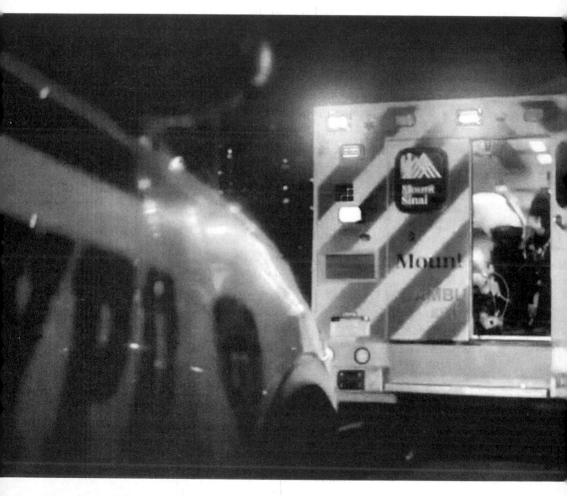

Mount Sinai treated and discharged 7,700 COVID-19 patients during New York City's first wave.
Previous page: ICU nurse Mereli Llarenas delivers care at Mount Sinai Brooklyn.

FEBRUARY 28, 2020—With much of the world still thinking the novel coronavirus existed only elsewhere, a Chilean named Rodrigo Saval was about to log nearly twelve thousand miles of international travel in just a few days. He was attending the annual ARCO contemporary art fair in Madrid, Spain, where he had been visiting family. He spent time with dear friends from Chile, who were themselves fresh in from the Venice Carnival in Italy. The carnival, which draws tens of thousands of visitors from around the world, had closed early as the first few cases of coronavirus popped up in what would become Europe's most devastated region. But at the time, many people believed the closing was out of an abundance of caution.

Mr. Saval flew home from Madrid to Santiago, and a day later would head off to New York, where he has an apartment. During his one-day layover, he felt fine as he visited with his parents, both in their eighties, his brother and his brother's eight children, and several work colleagues. As he got out of the shower and spritzed on his Jo Malone cologne, he noticed something odd: he had no sense of smell. Usually, he was "worse than a dog" when it came to olfactory sensitivity. He could tell who'd just come into a room by the waft of their perfume.

It was the middle of summer in Chile, and COVID-19 was on no one's radar. At age fifty-eight and a marathon runner, Mr. Saval felt hypochondriacal as he took his temperature before boarding a flight to New York—no fever—and felt run down as he landed at the airport ten and a half hours later. Chalking it up to jet lag, he lay down for a nap. When he awoke, he could barely breathe.

He dragged himself to a pharmacy to get a thermometer and struggled to convert its Fahrenheit to his Celsius, to understand if he had a fever. He did: 101 Fahrenheit. Friends urged him to go to the hospital, the nearest of which was Mount Sinai West, on Tenth Avenue near Lincoln Center, one of eight New York hospitals that, along with a leading medical school, make up the Mount Sinai Health System. Mr. Saval spent the night there in isolation, but, as protocol dictated at the time, he was sent home the next day to quarantine and await his test results. He didn't want to risk infecting a taxi driver, so he walked the four long city blocks to his apartment. "That felt to me like I was climbing the Himalayas," he recalled. "I couldn't breathe. It was so cold, and I felt, 'Okay, I'm going to die in New York. I'm going to drop dead on the sidewalk.'"

He spent an exhausting couple of days awaiting the results of his COVID-19 test, hearing from his brother in Santiago that their mother was not feeling well, and calling other friends and family he had recently been in contact with. He was in bed when he received a call on March 7, a "sergeant-like voice" from Mount Sinai, he said, informing him that he had tested positive for the novel coronavirus and should return to the hospital.

FEBRUARY 29, 2020—A week before Mr. Saval's test results came back, a married couple with respiratory symptoms came to the emergency department at the Mount Sinai Hospital, the health system's quaternary care center on the Upper East Side of Manhattan. The couple had just returned from Iran, which was one of the earliest countries to see spread of the virus beyond China and one that was on the United States' travel watch list.

New York State had just received authorization to test at its Wadsworth Laboratory in Albany—before that, COVID-19 testing could happen only at the Centers for Disease Control and Prevention (CDC) in Atlanta—and the city and state health departments had to approve each test. Gopi Patel, an epidemiologist and the hospital's medical director for infection prevention, began the call chain necessary at the time to get approval for COVID testing. She was told, "Please test for the novel coronavirus."

"It was completely life-changing," said Dr. Patel, who would soon become one of the public faces of Mount Sinai's pandemic response. She called members of the Health System's senior leadership saying, "I think this is real, I think this is it, I think it's here in New York."

If a health challenge was in New York, it was likely to be found at the Mount Sinai Health System—the largest in the city. The system has more than 4.5 million inpatient and outpatient visits each year across its eight hospitals and ambulatory clinics that dot the city and surrounding suburbs. Over the decades, Mount Sinai and its now 42,000+ employees had been a central part of the city's response to threats, including such epidemics as Ebola in 2014, H1N1 in 2009, and SARS 1 in 2003, as well as the physical and mental health fallout from the 9/11 attack on the World Trade Center in 2001. Among the health system's immutable principles were an overarching commitment to humane and compassionate clinical care, the practice and progress of social justice and equitable care for all, and the pursuit of biomedical research that makes a real and immediate difference in the lives of patients.

Now Mount Sinai was caring for the first patient in New York State and one of the first on American soil. Soon it would become one of the most essential health care systems in the U.S. COVID-response story. As the virus broadsided New York City with an earth-shattering virulence, Mount Sinai would find itself caring for thousands of COVID patients at the epicenter of the epicenter, across seven teeming hospitals. They included the Mount Sinai Hospital, which shared a campus with the medical school and was a nexus of advanced clinical care and groundbreaking science; two uptown hospitals across Central Park, Mount Sinai West, where Mr. Saval would seek care, and its sister hospital, Mount Sinai Morningside, serving the Harlem and Morningside Heights neighborhoods of immigrants, university students, and working families; Mount Sinai Beth Israel, downtown, which was at the time of the pandemic downsizing into a more nimble, outpatient facility; two outer-borough hospitals, Mount Sinai Brooklyn and Mount Sinai Queens, each with 200+ beds and soon revealed to be in the city's hardest-hit neighborhoods; and a new addition to the health system, Mount Sinai South Nassau on the South Shore of Long Island, still in the midst of integrating with the larger system but positioned to bring its patients the benefits of an academic medical center's advances in medicine and science—and not a moment too soon. An eighth hospital, New York Eye and Ear Infirmary of Mount Sinai, was not directly involved in coronavirus care.

Mount Sinai researchers, among the most prolific and best-funded anywhere, were well practiced in learning from the health system's enormous and diverse patient population and driving those scientific breakthroughs to clinical floors as quickly as possible. It would soon become clear that such integration was not only essential—it would need to be stepped up even further. The top-ranked Icahn School of Medicine at Mount Sinai had built one of the largest and most influential departments of microbiology in the country, with a specialty in influenza. As soon as SARS-CoV-2, the virus that causes COVID-19, was sequenced in January 2020, Mount Sinai researchers pivoted their work. This included virologists and scientists in many other areas, given the heterogeneity of this disease—immunology, cardiology, oncology, pathology, radiology, and pulmonology, among others—all fueled by an urgency to get discoveries to desperate clinicians and dying patients as soon as possible. Further, the academic medical center, with a robust clinical trials unit, would uphold its promise of early access to potentially life-saving drugs and would mobilize the clinical expertise to develop protocols in a whole new way, essentially in the fog of war.

ON FEBRUARY 29, the long, arduous journey had just begun. One of the leaders that Dr. Patel informed was David Reich, president and chief operating officer of the Mount Sinai Hospital and president of Mount Sinai Queens. He was at dinner that night with friends who were prominent members, coincidentally, of the Iranian community. When Dr. Patel reached him with the news, Dr. Reich returned to the table and suggested that his dinner companions cancel an upcoming gala in celebration of the Persian New Year.

He knew the world was about to change.

The next day, the COVID-19 test results came back for the couple seeking care at the Mount Sinai Hospital: positive for the wife, while the husband tested negative (although he was believed to have had the virus). New York State now had its first known COVID-positive patient. Suffering only mild symptoms and having followed proper isolation protocols, the couple quarantined at home.

A day after that, on March 2, Governor Andrew Cuomo said at a press conference, "Community spread is going to be real. That is inevitable."

And on March 3, a second case of COVID-19 would surface in New York when a man from suburban Westchester County tested positive for the virus after a labyrinthine search for care through other area hospitals. Tracing his recent footsteps, health officials investigated hundreds of recent contacts in his law firm, his synagogue, a local college campus, and hospitals where he sought care.

What Mount Sinai—the health system for one of the most global cities on Earth—had been preparing for indeed became very real. Protocols were pressure-tested. Anxiety rose to the fore. And people banded together to face a threat the likes of which no modern health care system had ever seen before. We had truly entered a feverish pandemic season.

"It was a very strange time," said Dr. Reich, who would soon be in several "huddles" each day to lead the hospital, as incident commander, and help steer the health system through wave after wave of a seemingly never-ending tsunami. "People felt very much out of sorts because life around them was changing in ways that were completely unexpected, and did so very abruptly—in both our personal lives and our professional lives. As we were adapting to this shock of the pandemic descending upon us, the realization set in that New York was caught completely unaware by massive community spread. People started showing up at our hospitals—first in the tens, then the hundreds and the thousands."

The figures would strain credulity if we were not all living through it, a pandemic that would strike more than 111 million people across the globe and kill nearly 2.5 million in its first year, not to mention shutting down global economies and constricting daily life to little more than house arrest. The United States led the terrible statistics, with nearly 28 million cases and more than 500,000 deaths from February 2020 to February 2021. Arriving de novo in New York City, COVID ripped through the metropolitan area and its hospitals with furious speed and virulence, with some 203,000 people testing COVID-positive in New York in the first three months of the pandemic, according to the CDC. For those whose condition was serious enough to warrant hospitalization, the fatality rate was a staggering 20 percent to 30 percent, an unbearable death rate in modern medicine.

MARCH 7, 2020—Governor Cuomo declared a State of Emergency in New York, expediting a series of processes and procurements to prepare the state for what appeared to be certainly coming its way. Twenty-one people aboard a cruise ship off the coast of California had just tested positive for COVID-19. The Mount Sinai Hospital opened its first isolation intensive care unit for anticipated COVID patients, ten beds, including four in negative-pressure rooms, and engineering efforts were being mobilized across the health system to build into the surge as needed.

It was a Saturday, and Judith Aberg, chief of infectious diseases for the Mount Sinai Health System, was heading to the Poconos with her family to take her granddaughter snow-tubing. On the road twenty minutes from the hill, Dr. Aberg got an emergency call from Don Boyce, vice president of emergency management, saying that Mount Sinai West was admitting the health system's first known COVID-positive inpatient, Mr. Saval.

Dr. Aberg is a thought leader in the field of infectious diseases and would very soon be at the heart of the health system's multifaceted clinical, operational, and scientific response to the pandemic. That Saturday, she asked for a few more hours, just enough for her granddaughter to have a quick slide before they returned home. She knew how onerous things were about to get.

"We knew it was coming, but we didn't know when it was going to hit," she said. "And, boy, let me tell you, my life has certainly changed since then. I'm of the generation that people say, 'Where were you when JFK was shot?' In retrospect now, I see how traumatic it was, that first call, because I can tell you exactly where I was and what I was doing."

Joseph Mathew, director of the intensive care unit about to receive Mr. Saval, can also tell you exactly where he was: at a conference in Chicago with other pulmonary critical care doctors, just days before Mount Sinai would curtail professional travel. Intensivists like

Dr. Mathew, who was an attending physician in the division of pulmonary, critical care, and sleep medicine, would quickly become the front lines of care for COVID patients.

"I was surrounded by intensivists from all over the country, and there was a lot of buzz about COVID. I was understanding what other hospitals were doing in terms of preparation, what is allowed in terms of taking care of COVID patients, do we do our normal critical care routine in terms of isolation, can we use devices like high-flow nasal cannula oxygen?" Dr. Mathew explained, describing a time of extraordinary national and global collaboration. "I got to learn what was happening at Johns Hopkins, at Northwell, at University of Chicago, in terms of their policies and procedures. I was able to bring a lot of that back to New York."

In addition to the hothouse exchange of ideas, there was also fear over the potential exchange of a highly infectious virus, an anxiety that would soon come to be shared by countless health care workers, indeed, by countless people around the world. *Is there someone in our group who is sick?* he and his colleagues worried. *How are we going to get home safely? What about the airplane ride?* "There was someone there with flu-like symptoms," he recalled, "which made all of us paranoid."

BACK IN NEW YORK, at Mr. Saval's midtown Manhattan apartment, emergency medical technicians arrived in full-body hazmat suits. They looked like astronauts, and Mr. Saval wondered if he was hallucinating. After the short ride to Mount Sinai West, he waited ... and waited ... in the ambulance bay. The hospital had a great deal of preparation to do to make sure staff was safe, spaces were appropriately sealed, and the proper protections and protocols were in place. To Mr. Saval, who goes by Rod and who has an impishly inviting sense of humor, the wait on a chilly March afternoon felt like a particularly punishing purgatory. He thought, "I'm not going to die from coronavirus, I'm going to freeze to death."

Inside the hospital, Raymonde Jean, a pulmonologist, got to work evaluating the patient. "This is a moment I will never forget," said

Dr. Jean. "There was a lot of anxiety that afternoon when we were called from the Emergency Room that we have a COVID-positive patient who will likely need to come to the ICU. I went downstairs myself to evaluate the patient, looking at his data and his chest X-ray. At that time, he was very stable, able to communicate very well." She feared that wouldn't last. Comparing the new X-ray to the one taken two days before, Dr. Jean saw a spread of hazy opacity in both lungs. "The disease had progressed significantly," she said.

Up on the eighth-floor ICU, staff gathered outside the double-chambered negative-pressure room that would become Mr. Saval's home away from home. They had done just-in-time training on donning and doffing personal protective equipment (PPE), the body armor of gowns, gloves, N95 masks, and face shields that would come to pervade the floors of hospitals—as well as the national imagination—in the days and weeks to come. Krystina Woods, who was the infectious diseases attending on service that Saturday as well as the infection prevention staff member on call, was on hand to make sure proper protocols were followed and protections taken. Beyond that, she wanted to quell the understandable anxiety of patients and staff in the face of this virus about which so little was known—except that it could spread silently and leave a lot of damage in its wake.

"Understandably, there were a lot of people who were really afraid," said Dr. Woods. "We had been reading all these headlines, we'd all been preparing. As much as you're mentally trying to prepare for it, there's nothing that can really prepare you for that moment when someone comes in.

"You don't know exactly how you're going to feel. For me, what I really wanted to do, in addition to supporting the staff, was to make him [Mr. Saval] feel that we were going to do the best we could for him," she continued. "I made it a point to welcome him to the unit, to introduce myself, to let him know that we would take the best care that we could of him."

The goal was to minimize contact with the patient while still meeting all his clinical needs—needs that clinicians didn't even fully understand yet. This virus was new. The dearth of information was remarkable for a clinical staff at one of the finest health systems in the world. So they did what they could. They suited up in proper PPE and assembled the medicines and supplies that the duty nurse would need to deliver care. *Plan ahead, gather what you need, minimize transit into and out of isolation rooms.* This was the rhythm frontline workers would come to know well in the coming months.

The receiving nurse was Amelita Cachuela, who goes by Amy. Her training, compassion, and faith rose to the fore. She sent a text to Dr. Mathew, at the Chicago conference: "I am getting a coronavirus patient on 4L/nasal cannula," she texted, including his prescription for assistive oxygen. "This is a test of faith for me. I need to be prayed up more this time."

"Hope you are doing ok, Amy," replied Dr. Mathew. "The patient is blessed to have you care for him."

"I am the blessed one to care for the patient," Ms. Cachuela texted. "The patient is here."

NONSTOP CARE ON THE FRONT LINES

'I could not get over how sustained the intensity was'

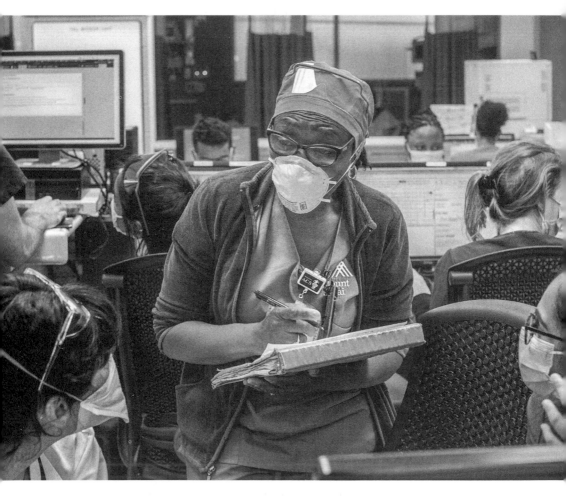

Marie Julien, assistant nurse manager, and coworkers navigate a busy emergency department at Mount Sinai Morningside.

AS THE DAYS WENT ON, a seriously ill Mr. Saval received dedicated bedside care from Mount Sinai West clinicians ensconced in personal protective equipment who were improvising ways to limit the number of people going in and out of his room.

Nurse Petra Cho would spend hours at a time in the negative-pressure room, "soaking," as she said, under layers of PPE.

Ms. Cho would write down what she needed, supplies and medications, and hold the list up to the window. The room, fortunately, had a sealed antechamber. Her colleagues would fulfill the requests, put the stock in the anteroom, then close the door, sealing the negative-pressure room back unto itself. Ms. Cho could retrieve supplies without exposing anyone else.

Ms. Cho felt a special connection to Mr. Saval. They shared the same birthday, February 22. Clinicians want to connect to their patients. With COVID patients often incapacitated or rapidly decompensating and family having to stay away, these modest human bonds would come to take on outsize meaning. Sharing a first name with a patient's daughter, discovering a mutual favorite song, being reminded of your own parents or grandparents. These threads would become part of the fabric of caring for patients during COVID.

Although Mr. Saval was intubated and sedated, Ms. Cho made breezy, reassuring conversation. "It's Tuesday today," she'd say, as she checked his lines and monitored his vitals. "You're in good hands here."

He was. As a leading academic medical center, Mount Sinai prided itself on ensuring that patients had access to the latest thinking and best therapies—a commitment amplified during the pandemic. Mr. Saval's journey provided a remarkable window into what was about to hit Mount Sinai, a cascading illness whose treatments were elusive and ever-changing. Clinicians, some of the best in the world, were in a terribly unusual position: not knowing the best course of treatment as their patients struggled for breath, for life.

Early on, it was unclear where, exactly, the virus was hiding, although Mount Sinai scientists were discovering important clues. Anxiety, on the other hand, wasn't hiding at all. It was front and center. PPE helped, and so did unprecedented levels of teamwork.

Working outside your scope to maximize patient care and minimize patient contact quickly became standard operating procedure. Neurosurgeons emptied trash. Plastic surgeons changed IVs. "Everyone," said one clinician, "was everything." That included stepping in as surrogate family members. With loved ones prohibited from visiting patients, clinicians in the midst of their hectic delivery of care—intubating, monitoring, rushing to code after code—took seriously their responsibility to ensure patients did not feel alone.

⁜

CARING FOR MR. SAVAL

'In early March, we had no evidence'

SHORTLY AFTER HIS ARRIVAL at Mount Sinai West, Mr. Saval had been put on a ventilator, a breathing tube threaded into the windpipe so the machine could fully take over that most basic primal act. He had WhatsApped his brother in Chile and the New York friends he'd deemed his health care proxies: "Guys, I'm being sedated and intubated. I'll be in touch in a few days."

But, as would be the case with many COVID patients on ventilators, Mr. Saval remained sedated and intubated—and unable to be in touch—for quite some time. Like so much else about COVID-19 interventions, the decision to put a struggling patient on mechanical ventilation was fraught, and clinical protocols would change many times over the coming months. But for now, the ventilator's setup—tubing went directly into the windpipe, creating a closed system—seemed a safer option than less invasive respiratory assistive devices, which could result in aerosolizing a patient's breath. And that breath was full of highly infectious virus.

"The news from around the country at the time was that it's better to intubate these patients early and put the endotracheal tube in, secure the airway, rather than take a risk with other devices like high-flow oxygen or noninvasive ventilation," said Dr. Mathew, speaking months later, having learned from the hundreds of patients he would go on to treat, as well as from the experiences of colleagues across the Mount Sinai Health System, the country, and the world. "So we intubated Mr. Saval as his respiratory status deteriorated. We had our anesthesia colleagues intubate him, which I'm sure was very nerve-wracking for them."

Beyond supportive care and intubation, advanced thinking in early March favored the use of the antiviral remdesivir, which was originally developed for Ebola and seemed to have some effect on SARS-CoV-2. The drug blocks one of the key enzymes that the virus needs to replicate RNA, which is how SARS-CoV-2 multiplies. While the drug was not yet approved by the U.S. Food and Drug Administration, it was possible to apply for it under the FDA's compassionate use policy, also called expanded access, which enables a patient with an imminently life-threatening condition to access medical treatments still under investigation if no other known therapies are available.

Erna Milunka Kojic, section chief of infectious diseases at Mount Sinai West and its sister hospital, Mount Sinai Morningside, was in frequent conversation with colleagues across New York City and the country and felt hopeful that remdesivir might hold promise for her new patient. Guided by Mount Sinai's commitment to get patients the latest treatments and well positioned to do so because of the relationships Mount Sinai had developed over the years through its robust clinical trials unit, Dr. Kojic moved bureaucratic mountains to give Mr. Saval a fighting chance. "If there's anything that will help besides symptomatic treatment, it is remdesivir, so I wanted to give this medication a try," said Dr. Kojic. "There's a lot of paperwork to apply for FDA compassionate use. It was really a group effort for all of us in the unit to get this for Mr. Saval."

Another challenge was to secure patient consent. As would come to be common during COVID-19, clinicians seeking patient or proxy consent for invasive or experimental treatments, as well as participation in clinical trials—all vital to advancing medicine and science—faced an uphill battle. Often patients were intubated or otherwise incapacitated, and the disease would come on so suddenly that families had no time to discuss contingencies. Further, as the pandemic went on, family members were barred from hospitals for their own safety.

But with visiting prohibitions not yet in place, a regular visitor outside Mr. Saval's room was his good friend Larry Wiesler, who, along with his spouse, Randy Federgreen, had been instrumental in getting Mr. Saval to the hospital in the first place and was serving as his health care proxy. In conversation with Mr. Saval's family, Mr. Wiesler consented to the treatment and praised Dr. Kojic for going above and beyond. "She said, 'I've been yelling and screaming, writing emails, not taking no for an answer—I'm getting this drug for your friend,'" Mr. Wiesler said. "She was so determined. It was impressive."

The course of severe COVID-19 was rarely linear, and shortly after his first doses of hard-won remdesivir, Mr. Saval's kidneys started failing. Back to Mr. Wiesler, to consent his friend for renal replacement therapy, or dialysis. That meant no more remdesivir, which was not recommended for patients on dialysis. "It was a roller coaster," said Mr. Wiesler.

For her part, Dr. Kojic described passing through stages of grief as a clinician, first confronting the novel virus with excitement, as an infectious diseases specialist who thrives on solving mysteries on behalf of patients. "It was new, and there was so much to learn about it," recalled Dr. Kojic, whose expertise had focused on HIV/AIDS and human papillomavirus (HPV). "Then it got worse, and we just kept seeing people do poorly and die from it. What started off as excitement turned into anger, followed by, frankly, just sadness. I definitely went through a grieving phase."

Dr. Mathew tried to look on the bright side, noting that even though Mr. Saval only got a couple doses of the antiviral, at least it had been introduced to his system. "We knew that it would prevent further replication of the virus," said Dr. Mathew.

COVID-19 HAD STILL more lines of attack in store. Early on in the pandemic, and borne out in Mr. Saval's case, clinicians realized that in many COVID patients, the immune system not only geared up to fight the invading virus but then, for some reason, went into overdrive, a condition initially referred to as a cytokine storm. Cytokines, inflammatory proteins, can be beneficial in fighting infection, but in abundance, they can overwhelm the body with inflammation, leading to organ failure.

Doctors tried an inflammation-blocking drug, to little apparent benefit. "We tried different things—remember, this was our first patient, and he was really not doing well at all," said Dr. Mathew. "After about a week and a half into his course—and I vividly remember this—we had a case conference with the other intensivists in our group, and we realized that, you know what? We have to do something different because whatever we're doing is not working. And we decided to give him steroids."

The decision was informed by conversations with colleagues across the Mount Sinai Health System, the city, and the country, as well as data that Charles Powell, system chief of pulmonology, critical care, and sleep medicine, had received from colleagues in China. The data from Wuhan's COVID-19 patients showed benefit from steroids, particularly in those with high levels of inflammatory markers. After weighing the mixed messages, Dr. Mathew moved forward. "On one hand, the WHO and others were saying not to give steroids because it prevents viral clearance," Dr. Mathew explained, referring to the World Health Organization. "But we knew that the standard critical care therapy we were doing for Mr. Saval, including lung-protective ventilation, dialysis, and so on, was really not working. So, we gave him steroids."

This, noted Dr. Aberg, was how treatments were navigated in those very early days of the surge, as clinicians were blindsided by a novel virus that continued to attack the human body in surprising and devastating ways. "Every day, we would have another observation," said Dr. Aberg. "We know steroids are approved for ARDS [adult respiratory distress syndrome, common in COVID-19 patients], and they're used for reactive airway disease. Also, our thinking was there is overwhelming inflammation, and steroids reduce inflammation. While steroids were not yet approved for COVID-19, they do have these other indications. Dr. Joe Mathew at Mount Sinai West advised, 'We're going to try this.' After a few patients are treated, he is in a position to say, 'Hey, I've now given several patients steroids, and it looks like they're doing better.'"

The steroids, in this case a treatment called methylprednisolone, worked to stabilize Mr. Saval's condition. At least for the time being.

Constant collaboration, relentless observation, and informed ingenuity were the orders of the day. Among the many experts Dr. Mathew and his colleagues were in touch with were those from the growing list of countries impacted by the pandemic. In addition to perusing the data from China, his team heard from physicians in hard-hit Italy, thanks to Mount Sinai fellows who invited them to weekly COVID case conferences.

"We were learning on the fly," Dr. Mathew reflected. "We try to practice evidence-based medicine, but unfortunately, in early March, we had no evidence. Ultimately, we realized, medicine is still an art. A lot of it is really dependent on what we notice works and what doesn't work."

÷

THE ANXIETY OF AN INVISIBLE ENEMY

'It's not just nursing, it's humanity'

THE RELATIVE LUXURY of having only one patient in the health system quickly came to an end. On March 8, a hospital transporter at Mount Sinai Morningside, Rafael Miranda, would mark his commitment to the health system's long COVID journey ahead with a simple disposable razor. Mount Sinai Morningside had just received its first suspected patient, and Mr. Miranda, along with his colleague Andre Cooper, was called upon to transport the patient from the Emergency Department to an inpatient unit.

But first, the men had to don protective N95 masks—and Mr. Miranda's could not be fitted snugly and securely over his beard. COVID-19 protocols were developing so quickly that many people had not yet been fit-tested for this level of PPE. "Without hesitation, he runs to the bathroom, shaves off his beard, throws on an N95 mask, and volunteers to move this patient," Mr. Miranda's supervisor, Rubiela Guzman, told *U.S. News & World Report*.

Then Mr. Miranda, clean-shaven and masked, did what he had done so many times before as a transporter, even as the clinical world around him was about to shift profoundly. Mr. Miranda wheeled the patient down the hallway, keeping the conversation light, as Ms. Guzman recalled, doing his best to mitigate everyone's mounting anxiety.

Anxiety was the byword of working on the front lines of a virus that was invisible, unpredictable, and deadly. There was no model, no manual, no clinical protocol for how to handle the spread of anxiety. Not even for a seasoned emergency medicine doc like Brendan Carr, who stepped into his role as the health system's chair of emergency medicine on February 1, 2020. Wasn't this kind of thing in his wheelhouse, as an emergency medicine expert used to fast-paced acute care? "Isn't this what you *do*?" he was asked.

"We do," he said. "Except usually the person we're taking care of isn't maybe going to kill us. We're not afraid of the blood. We can make fast decisions and do all the medical things we need to do. But facing our own mortality was never there before. In med school, they might say, 'Can you think quickly and multitask and stay calm under pressure and have no relationship with your patients beyond forty-five minutes or an hour, and still feel fulfilled?' But they don't add: 'And also be afraid every day when you go home that you're going to die.'"

Or get your family sick. Or lose loved ones yourself. Or colleagues.

"The hardest thing was managing fears," said Jennifer Jaromahum, deputy chief nursing officer at Mount Sinai West who took the night shift during the surge, while her husband and eight-year-old son slept. "It doesn't leave you after work. You're thinking of who you left at home, who you are going home to, and are you going to give it to them when you go home. But as long as our patients need us, we will go in. It's not just nursing, it's humanity."

Mount Sinai West's president, Evan Flatow, did his residency at the hospital when it was still Roosevelt Hospital, in the 1980s, at the height of the AIDS crisis. "There were thirty guys dying over here, and thirty guys dying over there," he said, gesturing from one side of an imaginary ward to another. As brutal as that epidemic was, COVID-19 was all the more transmissible, seemingly ubiquitous, and even capricious in its impact. Dr. Flatow is an orthopedic surgeon, not an infectious disease doctor, but he spoke for many clinicians when he said, "We accept risk—we don't shrink from it. But we're not soldiers. We don't *choose* risk. We're generally cautious people."

WITH THE FIRST two COVID-positive patients now admitted to the Mount Sinai Health System, changes both quotidian and profound happened in rapid succession. On March 9, when the Mount Sinai Hospital admitted its first known COVID-19 patient, Dr. Patel, speaking in an employee-wide virtual Town Hall, described the situation as "exquisitely dynamic." In short order, Mount Sinai would cancel gatherings of more than twenty people—lectures, events, meetings—then all in-person meetings of any size. Those who could were asked to work from home. "Do not shake hands," employees were advised. Social distancing was not yet recommended. Then it was.

COVID-19 was formally declared a pandemic on March 11. The World Health Organization's director general, Tedros Adhanom Ghebreyesus, tweeted that the WHO "is deeply concerned by the alarming levels of the coronavirus spread, severity & inaction, & expects to see the number of cases, deaths & affected countries climb even higher." On March 13, U.S. President Donald Trump declared the coronavirus a national emergency. That would also be the last day of in-person classes for New York City public school students for the 2019-2020 academic year.

Mount Sinai was now cancelling all non-urgent elective surgeries and medical procedures, to protect the public and to retain space and staff to treat the expected surge of COVID-19 patients. This decision would have financial repercussions as well an immediate impact on staff, many of whom saw their work disappear overnight and would soon find ways to redeploy to the vast COVID battle.

Meanwhile, many elements of the virus's spread and symptoms were still confounding. Health officials in all corners were racing to create protocols to mitigate infection and keep people safe. In a March 16 Town Hall, Dr. Patel told employees that it was unnecessary to require everyone to wear masks when they weren't providing care. The next day, mask-wearing became required for all onsite health care workers. In fall 2020, with the clarity of hindsight, Dr. Patel said, "I look back at that Town Hall and think, We said *what?*" She took a small degree of comfort in the fact that Anthony Fauci, the nation's top public-facing expert on COVID-19, was saying the same thing at the time.

No one yet saw all the places COVID was hiding. "In the early days of this, before we realized asymptomatic spread was such a thing, we were really careful with patients who had respiratory illness," said Dr. Carr. "But how about the guy down the hall, before it got really bad, who sprained his ankle playing basketball and gave the nurse and the doc COVID" because they treated him without pandemic-level PPE? "We weren't mindful yet."

He pointed to a meeting held in early March, documented in a photograph, in which more than a dozen members of the Mount Sinai leadership team convened in the Emergency Operations Center at Mount Sinai's 42nd Street administrative headquarters. The heads of emergency medicine, graduate medical education, supply chain, employee health, ambulatory care, information technology, support services, government affairs, human resources, key members of executive leadership. Shoulder to shoulder. No open windows. Not a mask in sight. "You saw us all in that command center," he said. "We're not wearing masks."

At the beginning of March, most clinicians, health care systems, and public officials were largely unaware of two crucial facts about COVID-19, which Mount Sinai researchers would soon discover:

- There was already robust community spread in New York City, which scientists would document by sequencing 90 genomes of the SARS-CoV-2 virus obtained from 84 COVID-positive patients seeking care at Mount Sinai between February 29 and March 18. In the journal *Science,* Harm Van Bakel, a genetic and genomic scientist, and his team determined that the virus had been circulating in New York weeks before the first diagnosis, and also traced New York City's COVID-19 outbreak directly to Europe, rather than Asia, as was originally thought.

- COVID-19 was not only a respiratory illness. Rather, its symptoms were maddeningly multifarious and could include strokes, blood clots, dizziness, loss of smell, and even no symptoms at all. This heterogeneity and the pathogenesis it suggested, hidden in the blood vessels, would soon be elucidated by Mount Sinai clinicians and researchers, including pathologists conducting a pivotal autopsy study of patients who had died of COVID-19.

╪

MONUMENTAL DECISIONS

'Oh, my God, we're in a war'

MARCH 17, 2020—The day would prove consequential for the Mount Sinai Health System. First, it completed validation studies and began performing SARS-CoV-2 tests in-house, rather than sending them to the New York City Public Health Laboratory or the Wadsworth Laboratory in Albany. That, said Dr. Reich, was a "game-changer." The process of seeking approval from New York City and New York State to conduct a test, then awaiting results, had become entirely too cumbersome now that there were hundreds of patients streaming into the health system. It could take up to six days to get test results, and, during that time, every "patient under investigation" was treated as COVID-positive. That meant, noted Dr. Reich, that "we were burning through PPE at a crazy rate."

The agility in testing meant clinicians learned the status of each COVID-suspected patient more quickly, could get the right patients to the right place at the right time—known as "cohorting"—and could wear the appropriate level of PPE without using up precious resources when they were not needed.

That same day, the Mount Sinai Hospital launched a 24/7 hotline to manage PPE resources ("we will have someone carry this phone around the clock," said the email notice). Behind the scenes, a vigilant hunt was on for protective equipment among skyrocketing need and a paralyzed global supply chain.

Also on March 17, Mount Sinai made an agonizing decision, one that would go on to deepen the tragedy of living and dying with COVID-19. Mount Sinai, soon joined by most other health systems in New York City and eventually around the country, decided it had no choice but to prohibit all hospital visitors, for their own, and everyone's, safety. It was a loss not only for families but also for clinicians, who counted family members as a vital part of the patient's health care team, of support, information, and follow-through.

The no-visitors policy felt inexorable at the time, amid such a transmissible virus whose bounds were not yet known. Just imagine if even more family and friends became involved in the spread. The consequences, however, proved deep and enduring. Isolation became an indelible feature of the COVID-19 story. Navigating the isolation as well as the disease would become an essential piece of the health care worker's job.

The decision reverberated throughout the hospitals, all the way to security personnel in the lobbies who were charged with turning visitors away. "That was an incredibly difficult task for the men and women of the security team to assume—to stand face to face with loving parents or a spouse or child of a patient who was dying and tell that person that they could not come in to be with their loved one, hold their hand, or express their love," said Timothy Burgunder, regional director of security. "They couldn't come much further than our front door."

TWO HUNDRED TWENTY-TWO COVID patients were being cared for across Mount Sinai's New York City hospitals on March 17, almost double the 115 patients from just two days earlier. "The floodgates opened," said Dr. Patel. It was not only the volume that overwhelmed clinicians. It was also the severity and unpredictability of the illness.

Madeline Hernandez, who had worked at Ground Zero after 9/11 and on a medical relief mission in Puerto Rico after Hurricane Maria, was the resus nurse on duty that day at Mount Sinai Morningside's emergency room. She was the team's point person to spring into action when a patient stopped breathing. Normally, any given shift might see a resuscitation or two. That day, Ms. Hernandez had five resuscitations at one time. "I was running from room to room to room, and I realized that it was almost already seven o'clock and the next shift came in," she told the Mount Sinai podcast *Road to Resilience*. "We didn't eat, we didn't drink, we didn't go to the bathroom. It was just nonstop."

Upstairs in the ICU, nurse Jessica Montanaro was caring for the first COVID-19 patient she could actually have a conversation with. Previous COVID patients came into the Surgical Trauma ICU, where she was assistant nursing care coordinator, already sedated, on mechanical ventilation, or otherwise too ill to communicate. But this man, Larry Kelly, was on a noninvasive breathing device, a BiPAP (bilevel positive airway pressure), taking in pressurized air through a mask to regulate his breathing. She fell for his outsize personality as soon as she met him. Although he was very sick, Mr. Kelly was awake and talking, his tan from a recent visit to Florida and his hale demeanor still perceptible behind the BiPAP mask. "A kind man, a strong man, I could just tell," she wrote in an email to the hospital's president, Arthur Gianelli.

But there was something heartbreaking in the way Mr. Kelly looked at her. "His eyes just looked terrified," she said.

She, too, was frightened of this disease, about which so little was known. She was in full PPE, following strict protocol, but because the patient was on a noninvasive breathing device, the air forced into and out of his struggling body seemed to swirl in the room around him. "It was immobilizing to me for a minute," Ms. Montanaro said. "That was the first time I realized I was truly vulnerable. We just knew nothing at that time. It was super terrifying. But I couldn't show him—I had to reassure him."

He kept asking her if she would help him breathe, a plea that went straight to her core. As a nurse, she was constitutionally wired to help. "You want to tell them yes," she says. "I did tell him yes."

But honestly, she wasn't sure. Even though Mount Sinai was one of the most accomplished health care systems in the world, with top-ranked clinicians and researchers and a staff dedicated to excellence, the lethality of COVID-19 was shaking the ground underfoot.

When Ms. Montanaro came in for her next shift two days later, she was stunned by what she saw. Mr. Kelly was hanging on for his life. He was intubated on very high oxygen requirements, hooked up to five IV drips, including blood pressure medication, a sedative, and a paralytic. "He was so ravaged so quickly," the nurse said. "He looked like some of our patients who had been here for three or four weeks with severe disease—and he was only here for two days. I was just promising two days ago that I'm going to help him breathe, and now we're *here*? I thought, 'Oh my God, we're in a war.'"

Describing herself as "the person who felt I needed to run into the war," Ms. Montanaro explained how everything she knew as a trauma nurse was tested during the surge. "As a critical care nurse, especially as a trauma nurse, you just don't get shocked by much, because we see so much devastation throughout our careers," she said. "But the level of shock that I was in every day I walked into that unit, it never went away." If she had left the hospital hours earlier, for a fitful night's sleep, the next morning a fresh shock hit her like an icy wind the minute she walked through the doors. "It was like getting hit in the face with just chaos. It was completely overwhelming."

MIRNA MOHANRAJ, a senior ICU physician at Mount Sinai Morningside, provided care to Mr. Kelly and scores of patients like him as the hospital, as she put it, "exploded." In the week from March 17 to March 24, the hospital's COVID patient census more than doubled—from 46 to 108—at the 495-bed hospital in the Morningside Heights neighborhood near Columbia University and the Cathedral of St. John the Divine.

Critical care doctors are used to exigency, but COVID-19 continued to outmaneuver. For highly trained experts used to saving lives through medicine and science, this level of uncertainty was new. "That's an uncomfortable place for a critical care physician like myself," said Dr. Mohanraj, who treated Mr. Kelly through myriad crises, including multiple seizures and brain hemorrhages as he clung to life for months. "We like order, we like control, we like having a plan ahead of time. With COVID, we were really having to develop clinical care plans that would rapidly evolve alongside similarly evolving infrastructure and organizational plans. Not only were we caring for an unknown disease, but we were also expanding our ICUs, managing new ICUs in places where we've never had ICUs before. It was an overwhelming, crazy experience. There are not a lot of other great words for it."

Furthermore, there was no end in sight to that intensity. Said Ms. Montanaro, whose husband would go on to contract COVID, "It wasn't like, 'Okay, this is a mass casualty incident and we're super-pressed in this short time.' It was just the everyday. I could not get over how sustained the intensity was."

Neither could David Reich, who had done considerable training in Incident Management, prepared for all manner of fire, flood, electrical failure, mass casualty events, and information technology disasters, all of which can have tremendous impact on patient care. But managing seemingly impossible clinical and operational hurdles day in and day out, for months and months, seemingly without end, was something else entirely. "Everyone was really, really exhausted— physically, emotionally," Dr. Reich said in an interview in September 2020, five months past New York's first wave but still very much in the midst of the pandemic. "Usually when a crisis ends, you have some sort of satisfaction. After the power failure, the power comes back on. After the snowstorm, the streets get shoveled. Humans need a beginning, a middle, and an end. Even if you don't like the way it wraps up, you want it wrapped up. But we never had that satisfaction."

‡

UNPRECEDENTED TEAMWORK

'Everyone was everything'

TIME COLLAPSED. Day blurred into night, March into April. Days of the week became unmoored. With more than 7,000 cases across the state, New York went on "PAUSE" March 22, mandating that all nonessential businesses close and all nonessential workers stay home. Mount Sinai's health care workers, of course, continued to come to work. They had hundreds, then thousands, of COVID patients to take care of. Emergencies—medical codes, cardiac arrests, intubations—happened with alarming frequency. At Mount Sinai Brooklyn, which with its community spread quickly became the most overwhelmed hospital in the health system, clinicians responded to 50 rapid response calls and 58 cardiac arrests in one 72-hour period, March 30-April 1.

At Mount Sinai Morningside, Dr. Mohanraj captured her days in cartoons doodled to help her process her experiences. One day, one cartoon—set on the sixth- and seventh-floor ICUs—stands out: "My cartoon for this particular day was, 'Run upstairs and do a code. Run downstairs and do an intubation. Run upstairs and do a procedure. Run downstairs and attend to this sick patient.' We were physically or mentally running all the time."

That "we" included everyone at Mount Sinai. "Not just critical care, really everyone in the whole hospital, the whole health system," Dr. Mohanraj emphasized. "It wasn't just doctors and nurses. Every hour of the day, our EHS [Environmental Health and Safety] staff was coming into the ICU and building new negative-pressure spaces while we were taking care of patients in that area. It was our administrators pulling together to help us figure out how we're going to safely open up a COVID ICU on a telemetry floor. It was every single person, our clerks, our cleaning staff—all of us learning together how to be safe and keep each other safe while still doing our best by the patients."

Putting people on ventilators—a significant and usually relatively infrequent procedure—had become harrowingly common. At the Mount Sinai Hospital, ventilator use quadrupled; at even harder-hit Mount Sinai Brooklyn, it quintupled.

Central to the battle for breath were respiratory therapists. "We're on all the code teams," said David Van De Carr, respiratory therapist at Mount Sinai Morningside. "We're experts in pulmonary medicine. We help people breathe, simply. It's the most important life function.

When you can't breathe, it's a desperate, desperate feeling. And that's what this disease is all about."

Mr. Van De Carr didn't watch the news about COVID as it overtook New York in March and April. As he said, "I'm living it at work. Our job is to go into COVID patients' rooms and put them on ventilators, get them off ventilators, put them on noninvasive ventilation. I go in and out of COVID patients' rooms all day. That's basically what's going on at the hospital right now. Everybody is COVID, and I see the worst of it. People there are very sick. Constantly throughout the day I have to choke back tears"—which he did, even in the retelling—"because it's overwhelming."

At Mount Sinai Queens, one day in April still makes ICU nurse Geneline Barayuga quake with emotion. She described rounding with the critical care team, which is par for the course as an ICU nurse. "Usually, we are looking at patients to see about discharge—*she can go home tomorrow*, or *this patient can go home at this time*," said Ms. Barayuga, her voice quivering. "But in April, we would go around the inpatient unit seeing which patients needed to be intubated. It was so scary that day, back-to-back-to-back intubation every ten, fifteen minutes. By noon, we had intubated eight patients."

Each time, she was mindful of the medical and emotional gravity of endotracheal intubation. "It's an uncomfortable procedure," she said. "You have to explain to them: 'We'll put you to sleep, and we might have to paralyze you so you don't feel anything.' They are very scared, and all they'll wish is for me to make a phone call to the mom or the family for them to say goodbye over FaceTime."

After the marathon morning, she went into a break room and threw herself into a chair. Her director asked her if she was all right. She answered, "It's too much. I've had enough. I don't think I can go on anymore." Through tears, she told her director about the eight intubations, took a moment, then got back to work.

"I still get emotional when I talk about it," Ms. Barayuga said in an interview six months later. Her husband, Nelson Barayuga, also worked at the hospital, in the laboratory department, and the two would drive to and from work together, often in stunned silence.

"I did it then," she said, "but thinking about it I wonder, *How did we go through it? How were we able to get through this pandemic?*"

The answer shone through in almost every story, every memory, every unwritten protocol and code of human conduct that came out of Mount Sinai at that time. The only way health care workers got through the pandemic was *together.*

Said Dr. Mohanraj, "We got through it as a team. When we needed to be lifted up, we lifted each other up. When we needed to carry someone, we carried them."

Jessica Montanaro was known as the "mom" of the ICU, and her Italian heritage drove her to make sure everyone had enough to eat. Bountiful food donations made that part of her job easy. Knowing the profound toll the work was taking on her colleagues, she conducted regular "emotional temperature checks." "That was a priority of mine as the clinical leader of ICU," she said, "to be aware of the staff around me and who needed what, and if they needed to get off the floor."

GONE WERE THE DAYS when medical emergencies were contained in certain parts of the hospital, to be handled by certain kinds of clinicians. At Mount Sinai Queens' emergency department, ED Nursing Senior Director Jonathan Nover explained that, typically, medical codes happen in resuscitation suites. They're designed for that, and they represent a small percentage of bed space in the emergency department. "But patients were just coding everywhere," he said. "Not just in our resuscitation suite—literally, everywhere. If you were rounding, or if you were responsible for a certain section, you'd start on one end and go patient to patient, then once you got back to the beginning, a lot had changed. It was so fast and so dramatic."

As a result, he said, everyone was working in unfamiliar territory—and more collaboratively than ever before. The need was urgent, and, with scant clinical expertise on this particular virus, everyone's insights and ingenuity were welcome. "The nurse's scope was definitely elevated," Mr. Nover said. "So was the respiratory therapist's, the physician's, the anesthesiologist's. There was a lot of critical thinking and action. Everyone was essentially everything in those situations."

People often worked outside their scope, too, to minimize the number of health care workers entering and exiting highly infectious spaces. Mount Sinai Queens Emergency Department had a motto: *If you go in for one task, complete ten.* "Help your colleagues to decrease exposure," explained Mr. Nover. "In situations where patients were coding, we had an intimate team managing those patients versus the traditional ten or twelve people getting in there to help. The staff worked very rapidly, but smartly."

At Mount Sinai Beth Israel, which was rapidly opening COVID units and reconfiguring workflows, Chief Nursing Officer Christine Mahoney said, "Everyone was playing their part, whether it was the part you were hired to do or not. Anybody would have done anything, pull trash, serve meals. There was no job that was not yours to own."

Nurse Montanaro recounted knocking on the door of a negative-pressure ICU room to get the attention of a redeployed neurosurgeon who was checking on a patient. The trash in the room needed emptying. It was safest and most efficient for someone already inside the room—i.e., the neurosurgeon—to do it. "So there he was, in PPE, changing garbage inside the room," said Ms. Montanaro, who communicated through a closed glass door many times. "There were no egos. We did whatever we had to do. We relied on each other and took on roles that we would have never done before. I wouldn't usually tell a physician to change my drip rate [on an IV]. But now I was standing outside rooms telling doctors, 'No, do this, change that, this is how you set up an a-line [arterial line].' We were all sharing each other's responsibilities."

One of those doctors was Mirna Mohanraj. "I learned how to operate pumps, and now I know how to do that," she said. "If I was in a room examining a patient, I didn't think it was right to call a nurse in just to change the sedative dosing. They trained me up to do that very fast."

She even learned to write backwards, so she could draft a list of needs directly on the inside of the window. "The rooms are really loud," she said of regular ICU rooms converted to negative-pressure COVID rooms via hose and HEPA (high-efficiency particulate air) filter, a now-familiar design solution to accommodate the surge. "You can barely hear each other in there, much less hear somebody who's outside."

Down at Mount Sinai West, Dr. Kojic not only checked in with clinical colleagues to see if there was anything else she could do while inside a COVID room. She also drew blood and nasal swabs for research teams at the medical school, closing entirely the distance between bench and bedside. Dr. Kojic had been working late one night when a woman holding a Whole Foods bag found her and had a request. "She asked, 'Can you get me lots of samples from this patient?'" recalled Dr. Kojic.

The visitor was Viviana Simon, a Mount Sinai virologist who since 2016 had been building a bridge between clinicians and researchers, the Mount Sinai Virology Initiative, whose mission was to prepare for the next pandemic by studying immune responses to viruses. While Dr. Simon (and many colleagues) had expected the next pandemic to be driven by an influenza variant, she quickly adapted her sample collection to SARS-CoV-2 from the COVID-positive patients just beginning to enter Mount Sinai hospitals. She wanted to collect blood and nasal swabs to sequence the virus, study the immune response, investigate antibodies, and explore whether the infection shifted to different cell populations, among other questions. "These were complete unknowns at the time," said Dr. Simon. Although her work focused on basic research in the Icahn School of Medicine's legendary microbiology department, she had trained in her native Germany as a physician-scientist and had always been impelled by science that impacts patients. (She joked that if you call her on her German cell phone, she can dispense medical advice.)

Dr. Simon returned to Mount Sinai West every day for the next fifteen days to pick up samples from Mr. Saval, code name "New York 2" (Mount Sinai's second patient). She would soon be collecting numerous samples as patients streamed into Mount Sinai hospitals. Compare this to her pre-COVID collection of severe influenza samples: ten to fifteen patients a year. "The scale was completely different," she marveled. "The sheer numbers were daunting and really, really scary. Those early weeks in March were truly mind-boggling." (Read more about the work of Dr. Simon and her virology colleagues, including details about immune response and virus spread, in Chapter 11.)

From the clinical floor, said Dr. Kojic, "I lost count of how many times I swabbed Mr. Saval's nose. These samples enabled our Sinai lab to develop ways to not just diagnose, but also treat and do the serology. Instead of waiting for us to get together, Dr. Simon just came there at night and found me. We truly crossed all barriers."

✢

ENSURING THAT NO ONE SUFFERS ALONE

'I just became a grandfather for the first time'

SINCE THE MARCH 17 VISITORS' BAN, one of the most devastating undercurrents of the pandemic was that people were isolated from loved ones in their final days and hours. Clinicians tried to deliver the familiarity of home, holding patients' hands and learning nicknames and family details so patients would feel known and loved.

Health care workers comforted, consoled, devoted themselves to patients as a family member would do. Yakira David, a second-year gastroenterology fellow, dashed out to a local drug store to get a patient denture adhesive when the hospital pharmacy ran out, so he could eat solid foods again. Mount Sinai West chaplain Donna Gormley performed a renewal of vows on a wedding anniversary for an ICU nurse and her husband, both sick with COVID, before he succumbed to the disease. Jessica Montanaro was caring for a young woman in the ICU, nineteen or twenty years old, about the same age as the nurse's daughter. The patient was struggling to breathe and terrified to be without her mother. Said the nurse, "I went in there and said, 'I'll be your mom today.'"

Health care workers kept cell phones and iPads charged and went from room to room connecting patients with family members via FaceTime and Zoom—often, to say goodbye. For one couple who couldn't be in the same room because one's COVID test was negative while the other's was positive, hospital staff held cell phones so husband and wife could talk to each other in their final moments together. When Mount Sinai Hospital ICU Nurse Valerie Burgos-Kneeland initiated a goodbye call for a patient and stepped away to give him privacy, he grabbed her hand. Health care workers were part of the family grieving process.

Pulmonologist Glen Chun phoned a patient's family to tell them their loved one wasn't going to make it and to request permission to remove the breathing tube. The patient's daughter asked the doctor to pass along a message to her father. So Dr. Chun went into the room, along with a nurse, and told the patient, "Your daughter loves you. She thinks you were the best person she has ever known. She cannot wait to see you in heaven."

Care providers captured as much personal information as they could on the glass doors and windows of each patient's negative-pressure COVID room. Picture the setup: closed door sealed against virus spread. Most medical equipment had been moved from inside the room to outside, meters of tubing snaking into the hallway so clinicians could monitor vital signs and equipment settings from there. Clinicians had taken to writing pertinent patient information right on the door, a kind of medical chart visible from the hallway. Blood value numbers, ventilator settings, lab tests ordered. Things like that.

And things like this: "I just became a grandfather for the first time and haven't met my grandson yet." And this: "My wife said I must come home soon to do laundry. She hasn't done it in 20 years." And this, as Camille Davis, a nurse at the Mount Sinai Hospital, told the *Los Angeles Times*: "The window to a patient's room said he had just had a grandbaby, and he loved R&B and had five grandchildren and four grown children, and he liked to go to Atlantic City." She felt so attached to his story that when his heart stopped and after extensive CPR, the attending doctor decided to call the death, "I said, 'Don't stop. Just one more,'" said nurse Davis. "That note made it impossible to stop." In the end, as so many gravely ill patients ultimately did in early

April, the grandfather of five died despite clinicians' tireless efforts.

Mount Sinai Morningside's ICU team accelerated a pilot project begun before COVID, the ICU Narrative Project, which asks questions of family members (or patients if they're awake) to capture personal life stories in a unit too often devoid of dignity and individuality. *Who are the most important people in your life? What are your most valued experiences?* And even, *What name do you go by?* The project had discovered, pre-COVID, that half of ICU patients prefer not the formal name on their medical record but a nickname or middle name. Clinicians learned that one of their COVID patients went by his middle name, which in his language meant "Bull" and conveyed strength. Said Dr. Mohanraj, who developed the pilot, "The craziest thing is that when we called him that, he was more responsive. I mean, it's not crazy. That's human nature."

÷

DEATH HITS CLOSE TO HOME

'What we endured together was difficult and painful'

AS CLINICIANS AND RESEARCHERS raced to get the upper hand on the virus, deaths mounted. In April 2020, 1,332 patients died across the health system. By contrast, a year earlier, in April 2019, there were 211 deaths. At the Mount Sinai Hospital, Joseph Herrera, head of rehabilitation and human performance, saw five deaths in a single day and, day after day, countless medical codes when patients' hearts stopped. "We thought we were going to see sick people for sure, and we thought we were going to make them better," said Dr. Herrera, who is usually focused on getting athletes (and the rest of us) back to peak performance. He didn't know that they would be scrambling to resuscitate patients who had stopped breathing, or pronouncing deaths. "That was something that we, I, did not foresee. We had a core belief that we could help."

This reframed—though never undermined—his understanding of the mission, of why he had repurposed his rehab unit as a COVID unit and his staff as COVID care providers. His team was guided by an unflinching principle: *If not us, who?* We're physicians, and there are not enough physicians to care for all these patients, he told his team, most of whom volunteered without hesitation. (The team had two other guiding principles: *Always don your PPE*. And, *Protect your colleagues, your staff, and the future*, meaning that the newest members of the team, the residents and fellows, would be the last to go into the riskiest situations.)

His colleague, Dayna McCarthy, who co-led the rehabilitation team, pointed out that their specialty, rehabilitative medicine, was founded in part to take care of World War II military veterans who no longer died of their injuries but rather had to learn to live with them. While the field was born out of war, she and her colleagues were used to coming in for the aftermath.

This time was different. Now, the physicians were coming in on the front lines. "I became a doctor to help when needed," she said. "I'm the kind of person where, if there's a battle, I want to charge in it. I hope I never have to see wartime medicine—but this was pretty close."

"WE HAD A LOT OF DEATHS," says Jennifer Jaromahum, who, as Mount Sinai West's deputy chief nursing officer, was the emotional and logistical heart of the ICU caring for Mr. Saval, among other units. "The nurses are not used to that much death, three or four times a day."

None reverberated more painfully than the early death of one of their own. On March 24, one of the most ebullient nurses on the eighth floor, forty-eight-year-old Kious Kelly, died of COVID-19, two weeks after testing positive for the virus and one week after being hospitalized. He was believed to be the first health care worker in New York City to succumb to the illness. Ms. Jaromahum still choked up when she talked about him, his spirit forever with her. He texted her while he was being intubated, and, in tears, his colleagues gathered on the eighth floor at the time to sing "Amazing Grace." Ms. Jaromahum still kept Mr. Kelly's white lab coat in her office, as well as his metal clipboard, which remained filled with the candy he was famous for dispensing to colleagues. When COVID set in and nurses were unsure of the disease's reach or wrath, Mr. Kelly, a nurse manager, used candy to cajole reluctant coworkers to join him in treating infected patients. "He'd say, 'Come on, we're nurses!'" Ms. Jaromahum said, infusing her voice with his energy. "He knew how much nurses could alleviate patient suffering."

His death was crushing to his team, said Ms. Jaromahum, and their grief-induced anger was captured by the New York media, which questioned whether health care workers had access to appropriate levels of PPE. Though guidelines were continually changing, and frontline workers were initially asked to keep N95 masks on for a full day—beyond the traditional single encounter/single use—Mount Sinai never did run out of protective equipment and took great pains to make sure it was on hand where and when it was needed.

"What we endured together was difficult and painful, especially losing our dearest Kious early on and receiving bad press," said Ms. Jaromahum. "But what we need to keep our eyes on is what more we can do for patients. Throughout, we've kept our focus on saving lives, conquering fears, and supporting each other."

The pandemic's death and destruction would become personal in other hospitals, as well, across the health system. Said Claudia Garcenot, chief nursing officer at one of the most embattled hospitals, Mount Sinai Brooklyn, "We lost a PCA [patient care assistant] and two doctors, including Dr. Dan [radiologist Sol Dan], who we were all very close to. We have staff who lost mothers and fathers. That doesn't happen with other diseases, right? Yeah, we know that people die from the flu, but how many people do I personally know who died from the flu? None. How many people do I personally know who died from COVID? A lot. A lot."

AS MARCH CAME TO A CLOSE, Rodrigo Saval continued on the COVID-19 roller coaster, a particularly cruel one that kept plunging down and down. He did not get better, indeed, he got much worse, but neither did he die. As days went by, 8AE 54, that first room in the ICU, became a touchstone of promise. Dr. Mathew's mother's prayer group kept Mr. Saval in their rotation. The health system initiated a daily moment of reflection and prayer at noon each day, called the Mount Sinai Miracle, and invited care providers, patients, and families to stop at noon to reflect and pray. Said Mr. Saval's friend, Larry Wiesler, "In Rod's greater circle of family and friends and friends of friends, there were on some days more than fifty people from literally all over the world reflecting and praying at the same time. The power of this initiative was tremendous—it created a common bond and solidified a community of care and purpose."

Dr. Flatow, Mount Sinai West's president, noted, "There's a lot of praying here. A lot of medicine and a lot of prayer."

"Rod became a mascot," said Ms. Jaromahum. "He was relatively young, healthy, he had run a marathon. He was someone everyone could relate to."

At the end of March, Dr. Mathew had to stop his hands-on care. He had gotten COVID himself. The case was not severe enough to warrant hospitalization, and he quarantined in the guest bedroom of his New Jersey home. His seven-year-old son, Evan, would leave a plate of food at the door for meals ("and then run," said his dad). Dr. Mathew continued to monitor Mr. Saval and other patients remotely—and harnessed reserves for what would still be the long fight ahead. "My stress level was so high," said Dr. Mathew. "I tell people that getting COVID is probably one of the best things that happened to me. It took me out of the hospital for a week, helped me get my bearings, and luckily I was able to come right back."

※

SEEKING TO HEAL THE HEALERS
'It takes a big toll'

ONCOLOGIST GABRIEL SARA was a young intern in his native Beirut when the Lebanese civil war was raging. He dodged bombs and bullets to treat the wounded, and he practiced medicine in a bombarded hospital basement, creating a makeshift operating room in a bathroom. "I had to become part of the resistance, not with weapons but helping people survive attacks by the Syrian army," he said.

Under siege in that hospital basement, Dr. Sara played his guitar and sang, first to distract people, then, because he saw it was therapeutic, to heal them.

Dr. Sara saw among the nurses he was working with now an emotional distress the breadth and depth of which he hadn't experienced since his days of war some four decades before. "Every nurse is overwhelmed *normally*," he explained. "Now they are in the middle of a hurricane that no one was quite prepared for." He praised nursing leadership for how they supported staff but noted that everyone needed another layer of support to heal.

"Think about a nurse's day during COVID," said Dr. Sara, who was known around the hospital for his generosity of spirit and commitment to holistic healing. "Each time they go into a room, they have to put on the gown, put on the mask, put on the gloves, put on the shield. Then coming out of the room, take off the gown, take off the mask, take off the gloves, take off the shield. Clean up, do it again. And each patient is a tragedy. Some are doing well one day, then the nurse finds out the next morning they died. Patients dying without family, a married couple dying in separate rooms of the hospital. Nurses held the phones so they could talk to each other as one died. Nurses were living this every day, and it takes a big toll."

Fifteen years ago, Dr. Sara created what has become known as Breakfast on 9A, a monthly healing meeting (think: food, music, and guided, though optional, conversation) for staff on the oncology floor. So he knew how valuable such sessions were, especially if they were embedded into the workday. Now, although groups could no longer gather in a room, Dr. Sara, in conjunction with Mount Sinai West chaplains and behavioral health experts, conducted daily healing sessions over Zoom and by phone. The key, he said, was to weave them into the course of a health care worker's day. He asked nurse managers to tell their staff, at the appointed hour, "*Stop working. Don't answer the phones. Someone's going to cover for you, so you can come take care of your mental health.*"

A carefully curated music playlist was essential. Dr. Sara described a particular session, attended by several Caribbean nurses and nursing assistants. "At the end of a very emotional session, I put on Bob Marley, and they were on fire—singing, dancing," he recalled. "It snatched the pain out of their chest."

"He understood early on the impact this pandemic would have on our mental health and had a vision of what the staff was going to need," Ms. Jaromahum said of Dr. Sara, adding that in her first session she "cried the whole time." "We'd go into those sessions and just unload. It definitely helped."

AMID THE CRUSH OF COVID CARE, health care workers could immerse themselves in another world, for at least a few minutes: the sun setting over a rippled ocean, snow-capped mountains descending into a glacial lake, a golden cove lapped with green waves and dotted with breeze-blown trees.

"Hey, Google, activate a lake," said an overworked Dayna McCarthy upon entering one of the twenty "recharge rooms" across Mount Sinai. Instantly, a tantalizingly realistic lake appeared on an all-encompassing screen, replete with an audibly crackling campfire in the foreground, birdsong, forest scents. She paused to breathe it in, took a moment of gratitude, and promptly fell asleep.

"I'm feeling really good right now," she said after her brief recharge, "and ready to go back to the floor."

Created by an environmental design company called Studio Elsewhere in partnership with Mount Sinai's Abilities Research Center, the research rooms transformed underused space—in hospitals or overflow tents—into oases of evidence-based calm. "We were hearing that our colleagues needed a place to decompress, to forget that they were in a hospital," said David Putrino, director of rehabilitation innovation who was the creative scientific mind behind the project.

Before the pandemic, Dr. Putrino and Studio Elsewhere had been developing a similar recharge space for high-performance athletes—NBA players—to help them accelerate their cool-down and recovery process. "When the pandemic hit," Dr. Putrino noted, "sports were not front of mind." In the span of about twenty-four hours, he and Mirelle Phillips of Studio Elsewhere pivoted their efforts to build out the first modular recharge rooms for health care workers. All the furnishings had to support the science of resilience and relaxation as well as meet hospitals' health standards. That meant including things like high-quality silk plants—antimicrobial and hypoallergenic—because research shows greenery is a physiological salve, but live plants do not meet protocol.

As a scientist, Dr. Putrino is guided by evidence, and his team published work showing there was a 60 percent reduction in self-reported stress levels after health care workers spent up to 15 minutes in one of the rooms. His ensuing studies would look at how the stress reduction translated beyond the moment, into workers' daily lives and performance of duties.

Mariam Zakhary, also a rehab doctor, described the deep and meaningful retreat to be found in the recharge rooms. "Every single thing around us was a negative statistic," she told *Wired* magazine. *"How many more lives were lost on our unit? How many ventilators short were we? How many more beds did we need out in Central Park? How much PPE did we have left?* But in the recharge room—for a few minutes, you weren't in that world anymore."

DAY IN AND DAY OUT seemingly without end, isolated in head-to-toe PPE and anxious about their own safety and that of their families, health care workers toiled in the borderlands between life and death. They could not even give an empathetic embrace, cry on a colleague's shoulder, or, on the occasion of a small victory, give a high five.

Dennis Charney, dean of Mount Sinai's Icahn School of Medicine, had his antennae up right away. A psychiatrist and expert on the science of resilience and PTSD, he knew the emotional and psychological toll of COVID-19 would be great. He had seen it before, in the extensive work that Mount Sinai had done with responders and survivors of the World Trade Center attacks on September 11, and in resilience research he had conducted with military veterans and POWs.

To calibrate the magnitude of need, Mount Sinai surveyed more than

2,000 employees at the height of the April surge. The numbers bore out the concern. Nearly 40 percent of the health care workers Mount Sinai surveyed were screening positive for risk of PTSD, depression, anxiety, or some combination. Almost half the workforce. In addition, the survey found that those who had been experiencing burnout before the pandemic were at greater risk of developing COVID-related PTSD. And, importantly, those who perceived higher levels of support from hospital leadership were at the lowest risk of suffering from PTSD, depression, or anxiety.

This was a clear message to health system leaders. "Mount Sinai's doctors, nurses, trainees, students, and clinicians and support staff are on the front lines of the battle against COVID-19, healing as many people as possible, yet they are witnessing death on a scale no one should ever have to endure," said Dean Charney. "Our health care providers are working at an intensity level so stressful that tens of thousands will likely suffer post-traumatic stress disorder in the wake of the pandemic. Their brave service ... is a debt we must repay through generous mental health support services."

To address that level of psychological fallout among health care workers, Mount Sinai—at the suggestion of a task force it had created—mobilized some eighty clinicians throughout the health system to provide mental health support to employees and students while still in the grips of the pandemic's first wave. Mount Sinai would go on to establish the Center for Stress, Resilience, and Personal Growth at the end of April, to monitor and mitigate health care workers' profound mental health repercussions and to train in resilience-building skills.

✢

HONORING EVERY DEATH

'You can't be numb to that. You can't.'

IN PRE-COVID TIMES, people facing a life-limiting illness might spend weeks, even months, having end-of-life conversations with their families about goals of care—deciding how far to push treatment in the final stages, weighing risk and quality-of-life implications. But with COVID-19, patients could go from being relatively comfortable to needing mechanical ventilation and facing end of life in a matter of hours. Furthermore, their families could not be present, and health care workers were stretched to their limit.

Never before had an entire hospital system (indeed, an entire planet) been in greater need of palliative care, a team-based specialty that provides an added layer of support for those with serious illness. One of the nation's leading experts in palliative medicine, R. Sean Morrison, and his Brookdale Department of Geriatrics and Palliative Medicine, quickly designed and deployed a telephonic help line to provide palliative support to clinicians and to patients and their families. Known as PATCH-24 (PAlliaTive Care Help), the line was staffed around the clock by Mount Sinai palliative care specialists and redeployed physicians, out-of-state palliative medicine physicians, and medical student volunteers. A PATCH-24 palliative care physician was also embedded in Mount Sinai emergency departments during the peak.

"This in-person presence in the fast-paced ED allowed for close collaboration in real time, where that palliative physician could meet with patients and families while the ED physicians triaged and stabilized patients," explained Dr. Morrison. "Palliative care physicians provided empathic listening and encouragement for frontline clinicians. They arranged for video visits with family, chaplaincy calls, child life specialists, art therapy support, and mindfulness coaching for families to not only support patients and families, but also to help distressed clinicians see the range of care that can be delivered even when death is imminent."

With so many very sick patients, all manner of clinicians ended up comforting patients at the end of life. Maria Duenas, a primary care doctor redeployed to a COVID unit, found herself having an end-of-life conversation with a longtime patient of hers now in the emergency room with oxygen levels below 60 percent when they should be in the high 90s. Dr. Duenas spoke the patient's native Spanish, but PPE created a whole new language barrier. Dr. Duenas painfully recalled "having to walk her through that goals-of-care discussion while wearing an N95 mask and face shield, wrapped in this gown and gloves. She's just sitting there, visibly panicked with this [oxygen] mask over her face just trying to take as many breaths as she can. It was the most challenging thing—you can only communicate with your eyes. It's the new COVID way."

Eyes locked on her longtime doctor, the patient said she did not want to be intubated, with the quality of life that likely conferred. Two days later, she passed away. "It was a very emotional conversation to be having in an emergency room in the peak of this crisis with a patient that I deeply cared for," said Dr. Duenas, adding that she cried long and hard when she got into a break room. "That whole experience will forever be with me."

Over at Mount Sinai Morningside, Dr. Mohanraj—PPE notwithstanding—felt an intense connection with a woman in her nineties who had just said goodbye to her family. The doctor and two colleagues were in gowns, gloves, masks, face shields. "If you had asked me six months ago, I would have said, 'God, that's horrible, to be shrouded like that and ushering someone through the end of their life,'" Dr. Mohanraj said. "But, you know, touch is touch, even if it's through a glove. I held her hand, we talked to her about her family's wishes for her, that they loved her, that she was leaving a mark on this world. She quietly passed away, then as a team we had a moment of silence, and we thanked her for allowing us to be a part of that important transition."

In Brooklyn, nurses paused after a death to bring to light a few human details. "They would just take a moment and say, 'Mr. So-and-So was someone's husband, or dad, or uncle, a baseball fan'—whatever it was that we knew about that person," said Claudia Garcenot. "As nurses, we know that everybody's a person, but this elevated it a step further—who they really were as a person. It closed their lives in a very positive way. If we gained nothing else, we gained the human side to dying and being sick."

At Mount Sinai West, redeployed physician assistants (PAs) and rehabilitation therapists, whose pre COVID work was on pause, volunteered to sit with patients in their final hours so no one would die alone. As part of the End of Life Companion Program, developed by Orthopedic PA Maureen Bellare, the redeployed staffers remained in a patient's room until he or she had died, holding a hand, playing favorite music, praying if appropriate, and connecting with family members over Zoom.

At Mount Sinai Queens, nurse Amparo Sullivan encouraged her colleagues to write a note to the family of patients they had cared for at life's end, so the family would know their loved one did not die alone. "This courageous woman wasn't just thinking about herself but was deeply concerned about how the pandemic was affecting us," the nurse wrote to one family. "Her bravery and thoughtfulness gave me inspiration." Other notes read: "Your mother was in no distress when she passed peacefully. I spoke to her and told her how much her family loves her." "Your father was so, so brave. I won't forget him." "People show you who they are down to the core when they are in life-and-death situations. Your mother was so kind. I prayed for her on my lunch break."

"We hope it will give them a little peace of mind," Ms. Sullivan said of the families. "And it's therapeutic for us."

Mount Sinai hospitals, like many hospitals, are committed to healing body, mind, and spirit. An important part of the health care team, hospital chaplains provide spiritual care and comfort across faiths and traditions. During COVID, their role was amplified, as they worked long hours to bring comfort to the living and the dying in greater volume than ever before.

As the sole chaplain at Mount Sinai Queens, the Rev. Rachelle Zazzu performed dozens of bedside memorials in one seventy-two-hour period, including for those in a morgue truck parked outside the hospital. "These are not *patients*, these are *people*," said Dr. Zazzu, who worked twenty-three days in a row during the surge. "And on the other end of the FaceTime call is their daughter, son, husband, or mother who last saw them when they were a little short of breath and had a fever, and now they will never see them again. Ever. The only one who will sing their name to God is me. You can't be numb to that. You can't."

Dr. Zazzu described what it was like to hold a bedside memorial service—although it was too risky to be at the actual bedside, so she stood in a corridor—in the middle of a pandemic:

> There's a bed alarm going with the rush of four people saying, 'Manpower in 604,' while you're hearing 'Rapid response in 318,' and people rushing by you to get there, while you're hearing paging that someone's on the way into the emergency room. And that's very often happening while I have my hands on a door doing the bedside memorial.
>
> I'm outside a room, and I'm in full-on PPE, bonnet, goggles, shield, N95, scrubs, gowns, gloves, booties, with a family on FaceTime, which I have facing into the room where they can see their deceased loved one. They can see a mound with a sheet over it, or they can see the white body bag. I'm singing this person's name to God—Buddha, Allah, Mohammed, Christ, or Jehovah—and I'm saying whatever prayers are appropriate for that family with my hands on the door.
>
> Then I'm quiet and I ask them if they want to speak to their father, mother, son, daughter, brother, sister. I say, 'I don't care what the world is doing. Right now, we're not in a rush. Right now, you are the only thing that matters.'
>
> Whenever that's done, I go on to the next one for the next family.

Dr. Zazzu also strived to bring comfort to her colleagues, whisking them into the stairwell for a "meeting" away from the crowded hallways or making her presence felt to lighten the heaviness. "I just did everything to make them laugh," she said. "I told the most ridiculous jokes, and I would sing—I mean this literally—at the top of my lungs. *Rise and shine and give God your glory, glory.* Just keep in mind all the doors are closed and there's no visitors, right? And they would be like, 'Oh, honey, don't quit your day job.' But they would laugh."

She did more than tell bad jokes and sing out loud. She exalted her colleagues—and exalts them still, every chance she gets. "People will never understand the magnitude of what these health care workers sacrificed to come to work every day during COVID. It's superhuman. Talk about, 'Lay up your treasures in the kingdom of heaven,'" she marveled, quoting from the Book of Matthew. "Whatever spotlight you can, shine on them. Honor them, exalt them."

3 | ADVANCING PROTOCOLS

'Spark of light and hope'

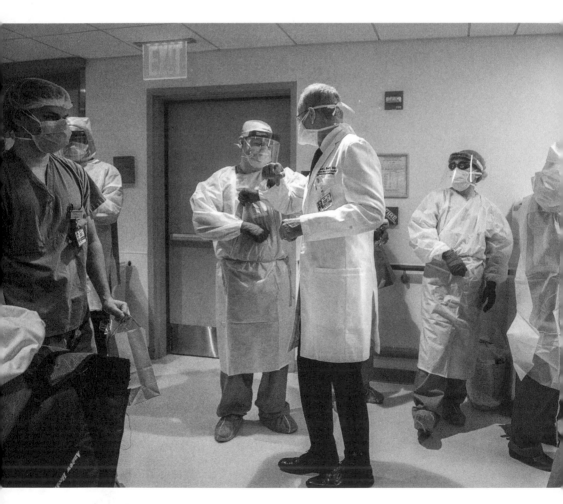

David Reich (center), president of the Mount Sinai Hospital, was everywhere during the surge, on the floors of the hospital, in huddles, and meeting with local and national health officials.

We had no known therapies. How do you treat individuals when there's nothing there to treat them with?

—JUDITH ABERG, *chief of infectious diseases, Mount Sinai Health System*

———

MARCH 28, 2020—New Yorkers had just started throwing open their windows at 7 p.m. to cheer health care workers, a rallying cry that would last throughout the spring. The first national CARES Act, the $2.2 trillion economic stimulus package, had just been signed into law. Mount Sinai was caring for more than 1,000 COVID patients—an alarming number that was about to climb by 50 percent in the next week, to near-peak.

The health system and New York City were still on the upslope of a frightening hospitalization curve when a ray of hope came to the COVID wards in a humble, unassuming package: a bag of golden liquid that could be transfused like a common blood product.

In a grand collaboration between clinicians and scientists, between health care workers and the New York community, Mount Sinai became one of the very first hospitals in the United States to transfuse patients with convalescent plasma, purified blood rich in antibodies from now-healthy people recently recovered from COVID-19. In the right patients, at the right time, clinicians began to see benefit from this treatment—at a time when they had precious else to offer patients beyond supportive care. "Just that glimmer of, 'We can come up with something to beat this'—that was an emotional boost," said Vicki LoPachin, Mount Sinai's chief medical officer and one of the health system's four-member Emergency Operations Center Unified Command Group. "It's that little spark of hope and light."

In addition to the convalescent plasma program, Mount Sinai clinicians also rapidly developed and disseminated a protocol to combat life-threatening blood-clotting in COVID patients. And they scaled throughout the health system a technique called proning, repositioning intubated patients on their stomachs to ease pressure on the lungs and help them breathe.

Make no mistake—these were not cures. Patients were still

decompensating and dying at terrible rates, first in New York City and soon around the country. But with Mount Sinai and New York City broadsided by the volume and virulence of the virus and a glaring lack of clinical guidance, these modest advancements— convalescent plasma, anticoagulation, and proning—implemented in record time, gave patients, families, and health care workers that glimmer of hope.

÷

CONVALESCENT PLASMA
'A shot of energy'

CONVALESCENT PLASMA was a nineteenth-century idea repurposed for a twenty-first-century pandemic. In the 1890s, the German scientist Emil von Behring successfully treated diphtheria in humans with convalescent plasma from infected horses, a breakthrough that earned him the Nobel Prize. More recently, doctors have used the antibody-rich plasma from patients to treat a modern era's new infectious diseases, including the first SARS virus (SARS-CoV-1) and H1N1.

The idea is that a body that has contracted a communicable disease, in this case COVID-19, musters antibodies to fight the invader, and those antibodies remain in the bloodstream even after someone has recovered from illness. Take that blood, separate out the red blood cells to leave the antibody-rich plasma, and transfuse the plasma into a sick patient who has not yet made enough antibodies of his or her own to mount a winning fight. This creates a "passive" immunity thought to persist for several weeks, in contrast to vaccines, which create active immunity that lasts for months or years.

To make the transfusions pay off, you want the plasma from people with high levels, or high titers, of antibodies. Mount Sinai was in a unique position to know the level of antibodies any potential donor had produced because of a serologic test developed right out of the gate by one of its star virologists, Florian Krammer. His assay was the first that not only determined whether someone had antibodies to the novel coronavirus but also quantified the level of antibodies—enabling Mount Sinai to screen for the desired high-titer plasma.

Judith Aberg, who had been involved with the National Institutes of Health's convalescent plasma collection during the H1N1 outbreak in 2009, was emailing and conferring with colleagues from those days about reviving such a program. On a March 23 national teleconference with the FDA and national experts on convalescent plasma, Dr. Aberg and David Reich urged action on the experimental treatment. Patient admissions were doubling every three days in New York City. By the next day, the FDA had posted on its website an emergency investigational new drug (eIND) program to permit convalescent plasma transfusion. The eIND program, often called "compassionate use," serves patients gravely ill from a disease with no known treatment.

Mount Sinai moved fast. On March 25, Dr. LoPachin sent an email to Mount Sinai's 42,000 employees asking those who had recently recovered from COVID to consider having their blood screened and, if appropriate, becoming donors. The request, noted Dr. Reich, "went a little viral." Thousands responded, although not everyone was a qualified donor. In fact, not everyone had even had the disease. But people were so eager to help.

In notes he kept to document Mount Sinai's many extraordinary COVID stories, Dr. Reich described the hothouse effort behind the plasma collection program:

> Florian's post-doctoral trainees, the Hospital Laboratory team, and a small army of information technology experts collaborated seamlessly in the middle of March to find equipment and reagents, and establish computer interfaces to the electronic health record systems. Another team set up a clinic for blood draws and nasal swabbing to test recovered patients. And yet another group, this one including our intrepid medical students, created a social media outreach to recovered patients, scheduling them for antibody testing, tracking their results, then scheduling the patients to donate convalescent plasma. This all happened in one week in late March.

WORD ALSO SPREAD through the Westchester communities that were hit in early March. Danny Riemer, a thirty-seven-year-old from one of those communities, New Rochelle, New York, was one of the first recovered patients to donate. "I think that for people who have recovered from the virus and are thinking about what they could do to help, this is probably the least heroic way possible to be a hero," Riemer told NBC News. "It's almost as if a survivor is able to pass the life raft on to the next person who needs it."

By March 28, the first patient received convalescent plasma at the Mount Sinai Hospital.

Under the FDA's eIND program, Mount Sinai had to apply separately for each patient it planned to transfuse. The FDA would review, then approve or deny each application. While the application process was laborious, the speed from idea to transfusion was head-spinning. Rather than implementing a traditional training period for a new clinical procedure, the convalescent plasma team walked the nurses through the process in real time, over the phone, framing it in a familiar context: *Deliver the plasma as you would any other blood product.* Nurses had had plenty of experience delivering blood products. Nicole Bouvier, a microbiologist and infectious diseases doctor who was the convalescent plasma program's principal investigator, did her best to explain what convalescent plasma was, why they were using it, and what the hope was for the patient.

"There was a lot of education on the fly, which we couldn't do ahead of time because there was no *ahead of time*," said Dr. Bouvier, who ran the trial alongside her counterpart on the plasma-collection side, Ania Wajnberg, as well as Dr. Aberg. Dr. Bouvier was primarily a basic researcher and part-time clinician who, in the way duties realigned during the surge, was now in charge of her first IND protocol. Her lack of experience with the bureaucratic ins and outs that she was up against (and soon had experienced hands to help with) may have actually helped her undertake the seemingly impossible, setting up a program of this magnitude in the span of days rather than months.

The key to convalescent plasma's success was in the timing of the transfusion. To gain benefit, hospitalized patients had to be transfused early in their course, before they began making their own antibodies and before they, as Dr. Bouvier put it, "went off a medical cliff," which is to say, needed mechanical ventilation or began to go into organ failure. "At that point the horse had already left the barn," she said. "What we were trying to do was catch people who looked like they were moving in a bad direction but hadn't quite gotten there yet."

One patient in that treatment window was Claudia Garcenot, who had been caring for COVID patients in her overrun hospital before getting sick herself. Now she was hospitalized with COVID at the Mount Sinai Hospital in Manhattan and was asked if she wanted to receive convalescent plasma. She knew it was considered experimental, but she felt so sick that the choice was clear. "I think if they had said to me you have to stand on your head for three days, I probably would have tried that," she said.

Two units of plasma and forty-eight hours later, Ms. Garcenot was on the road to recovery, crediting the treatment as the turning point. By the time she returned to work, she felt so strong and healthy that she joked, "I really think if I got plasma maybe three times a year, I would feel extraordinary."

Mount Sinai South Nassau was quick to bring the experimental treatment to its Long Island community. The night of the first delivery fell during Passover. Aaron Glatt, chief of infectious diseases and chair of the department of medicine at MSSN, walked five-and-a-half miles, each way, from his home to the hospital, since he, as an observant Jew, could not drive on the holiday. "I felt it was important that I come in, but don't focus on that, because there were so many people who came in for an unimaginable amount of hours of work," said Dr. Glatt, who had never before come into work on Jewish holidays. "The important thing to focus on is that with Sinai, we were one of the first places to do antibody testing in our community. We tested about 1,500 people, mostly from Long Island's Five Towns, who'd had COVID, to see if they would be eligible donors. We had zero proven medications to treat COVID, and this was a tremendous community, hospital, and systemwide effort to make this hopefully good treatment available."

One South Nassau COVID patient, Jennifer Woodard, was suffering from double pneumonia. Her lungs, she said, felt stuck with a hot poker. Even on supplemental oxygen, the 45-year-old Long Island mom struggled to breathe and had trouble getting out of bed. Then she received an infusion of convalescent plasma. By the next day, she said she felt like she had been given a "shot of energy." She required less oxygen, both in bed and while walking. "I am young and have a young family, and I couldn't fathom the idea of going on a ventilator," she said.

The treatment was a shot of energy, too, to health care workers. "It was definitely a positive for our staff, the frontline providers who were just getting pummeled and had very little hope at that moment," said Dr. Bouvier. "In the early days there was literally nothing you could do. And it's human desire to do something."

FOR PATIENTS who received plasma at the right time in their hospitalization, the outcomes appeared positive. In an early study, researchers compared the first 39 patients treated with convalescent plasma to similar hospitalized patients who did not receive the plasma. Researchers matched as many variables as they could, including age and underlying conditions as well as treatment with certain other medications, intubation status and duration, length of hospitalization before transfusion, and oxygen requirement on day of transfusion. "The final data showed that we did what we were trying to do and that it seemed to confer some benefit in terms of getting people off oxygen and getting them out of the hospital alive," said Dr. Bouvier.

In results published in *Nature Medicine*, the study found that by the program's conclusion on May 1, 12.8 percent of convalescent plasma recipients died, compared to 24.4 percent of the matched control patients. In addition, 71.8 percent of plasma recipients were discharged from the hospital alive, while 66.7 percent of the non-recipients were. "Overall," said the authors, "survival probability was greater in convalescent plasma recipients than controls."

In publishing retrospectively about the program—whose primary purpose was urgent, compassionate-use treatment, not research—the authors noted that they could not rule out other factors in the improvement. For instance, as the *Nature Medicine* paper noted, "We cannot exclude the possibility that convalescent plasma recipients benefited from generally more assertive clinical management by their primary physician teams."

But in the heat of battle in late March and early April, something safe and modestly effective was better than nothing, and the relative success of this new treatment option lifted the spirits of health care workers, patients, families, and recovered patients seeking a way to help. By mid May, with New York City's first wave on the wane, Mount Sinai had transfused 400 patients with convalescent plasma.

Said the *Nature Medicine* paper's first author, medicine professor Sean Liu, "As we face one of the largest pandemics of mankind, physicians and scientists will continue to unite in our common interests to return to a safe, normal life. It's not easy, but this is a step forward."

✣

ANTICOAGULATION PROTOCOL

'It took days, not years'

AS RODRIGO SAVAL went from bad to worse at Mount Sinai West, from ventilation and remdesivir to multiorgan failure and dialysis, clinicians noticed something alarming in his dialysis tubing: tiny blood clots clogging the catheters. He was, as clinicians say, "clotting out."

"That was one of the earliest signs that told us that COVID-19 patients are very prone to clotting, to develop clots in their legs, which could potentially go to the lung," said Dr. Mathew, referring to not only Mr. Saval but many early patients.

At Mount Sinai Queens, the first patient that Kathy Navid, acting chief of medicine, treated was a young man whose condition plummeted suddenly and vertiginously. "He fell off a cliff," she recalled. "I thought, 'Why is this young guy clotting?'"

Over at the Mount Sinai Hospital, Hooman Poor, an ICU doctor and assistant professor of medicine, ducked into the office of his colleague, Charles Powell. "I think I solved COVID!" Dr. Poor exclaimed, describing a significant finding he had just made. Dr. Poor, who literally wrote the book on mechanical ventilation (*Basics of Mechanical Ventilation*), had been finding that patients with COVID-19 did not have typical pneumonias. For one, their lungs were not stiff. This and other markers indicated that the lungs were receiving air but the blood flow to the lungs was blocked—evidence of clotting. (This would later be confirmed by a major autopsy study out of Mount Sinai's pathology department, one of the largest during the pandemic, which showed the virus attacked the lining of the blood vessels, the endothelial cells, and led to clots large and small.)

J Mocco, director of Mount Sinai's program that treats strokes by removing clots in arteries to the brain, had been noticing more stroke cases at the end of March. He became convinced of the problem on April 2, when he had four simultaneous cases in younger patients at very low risk of stroke—but who had COVID. "This was a bit of an alarm for all of us," Dr. Mocco told NPR after publishing a piece in the *New England Journal of Medicine* identifying large-vessel stroke as a "presenting feature" of COVID in relatively young adults. "We saw a sevenfold increase in the number of patients in their 30s and 40s who were presenting with severe strokes. And those patients did not have many of the typical risk factors we worry about for stroke. This immediately alerted us that it's likely the disease has a component that's causing clots and potentially putting people at increased [risk of] stroke but also other diseases caused by clots—renal failure, heart attacks, and other things."

Dr. Mocco ran into David Reich in the corridors of the hospital and told him about the alarming findings. "Talk to Hooman," Dr. Reich suggested, believing that the two men would come up with something together even greater than the sum of their individual findings.

At the same time, intensive care physician Sanam Ahmed also stopped Dr. Reich in the hallway (during the spring surge, Dr. Reich seemed to be everywhere, always present on the floors, in huddles, speaking with local and national governing bodies and media about

New York City's experience and Mount Sinai's response—and responsibility). Dr. Ahmed talked to him about the excessive clotting she'd noticed in the IV lines of COVID patients. She wanted to start them on anticoagulants, blood thinners that break up the clotting. But Dr. Reich believed the decision to offer this treatment should be an iterative process, something that was developed as a team and standardized across the system. That was soon—very soon—to come.

Since mid-March, Valentin Fuster, one of the world's leading cardiologists and the director of Mount Sinai Heart, had also been noticing patients developing blood clots in the leg. That observation—in conjunction with the brutal mortality rate and early papers out of China suggesting blood clots were associated with COVID—convinced Dr. Fuster, who has more than fifty years' experience in cardiology, of the best way forward: "Everybody should be on anticoagulation," he said, meaning all COVID patients admitted to the hospital (with other risk factors taken into consideration). "This was an intuitive feeling I had, that this would be important to the outcome of these patients. I have been in the business of clotting for all my life. This was a new disease, but certainly there were clots."

Dr. Fuster, along with colleagues William Oh, chief of hematology/oncology, and Andrew Dunn, chief of hospital medicine, began drafting a protocol to guide Mount Sinai clinicians on how, when, and in what types and doses to deliver anticoagulants to COVID patients. The team updated colleagues in the many system and department huddles held throughout the day, including the leadership huddle each day at 7:30 a.m.

What happened next—in the normally slow-moving world of health care bureaucracy—was remarkable. Within ten days from start to finish, a new clinical protocol was being rolled out across seven Mount Sinai hospitals. "Anticoagulation was another of those aha moments, offering a glimmer of hope that we can figure something out, we can help beat this disease and decrease the rate of death that we were all seeing," said Dr. LoPachin, who, in her role as CMO, was responsible for ensuring quality and safety across the health system. "I had the anticoagulation protocol agreed upon, put through everybody's P&T [pharmacy and therapeutics] committee, and implemented into an order set in the electronic medical record in less than two weeks."

Before COVID, she said, "That would have taken me about a year and a half."

That meant that promising anticoagulant treatment would immediately benefit patients not only in the major Manhattan hospitals but also out in Queens, Brooklyn, and the South Shore of Long Island, where the need was great.

Cameron Hernandez, who became executive director of Mount Sinai Queens during the pandemic, marveled at how rapidly a collaborative team could move from observation to action—crucial for Queens doctors who were, as he said, "running around at the height of this craziness with a gazillion patients." Said Dr. Hernandez, "With a team approach, we learned things quickly. People were talking about it throughout the system. *We're clotting off all the dialysis machines. We need anticoagulation.* Literally within days, we had a whole anticoagulation pathway here: what people get, who gets it, when they get it, who should give it. And it took days, not years."

Certainly Warnell Vega would not have had years to wait. The thirty-three-year-old Harlem resident, who was quarantining with suspected COVID, had been rushed to Mount Sinai Morningside when he collapsed at home and his mother called 911. He indeed tested positive for COVID and was admitted to the ICU, where doctors discovered a large clot blocking a lung artery. He was immediately started on the anticoagulation protocol, among other medications.

"He was really in dire straits," his doctor, John Puskas, site chair of cardiovascular surgery, told NBC news. "The clot almost completely blocked blood flow to his right and his left lungs."

As Mr. Vega lay in bed, on assistive oxygen but not a ventilator, he listened to the loud humming of the hospital around him and was grateful to be alive. "I know what the doctors tried was something new," said Mr. Vega, who continued to take two blood thinners, including low-dose aspirin, once he returned home to his fourth-floor walk-up. "They did a great job."

CALLING THE anticoagulation protocol "empirical therapy," Dr. Reich made a distinction between what physicians are used to—data-driven, carefully researched protocols—and what COVID had wrought. "We made clinical observations, then we reacted by creating what was a reasonable protocol at that moment in time," he said.

When Dr. Powell gave a view-from-the-frontlines talk to the American Thoracic Society in the spring, to colleagues specializing in diseases of the lung, he highlighted anticoagulation as a centerpiece of Mount Sinai's early COVID response (informed by the Wuhan experience, as well). There was pushback, he noted, from those not yet in pandemic hotspots who believed "there wasn't sufficient data available to be more liberal with anticoagulation." True, Dr. Powell acknowledged. But he added, "There wasn't data because it's all new. There was, however, enough evidence in front of us, accumulating very quickly, to demonstrate that clotting was a prominent pathophysiological phenomenon of this disease that was associated with morbidity and mortality." In other words, blood clots were killing people, and doctors had to act fast.

Physicians under siege in Wuhan, and then those in New York City, did not have the luxury of clinical trials yet. "All of us consider ourselves to be data-driven and like to be prudent about how we approach clinical problems and research questions," said Dr. Powell, who is a well-regarded expert in lung cancer and directs Mount Sinai's partnership with the National Jewish Health Respiratory Institute. "There are some situations where you just don't have the data. Rely upon your instinct and experiences and carefully track how your interventions are working while awaiting results of definitive clinical studies."

Doctors were essentially stamping out fires, with people crashing and dying around them. Once they could look up, once there was time, they would undertake rigorous research into COVID-19's impact on the cardiovascular system and how to mitigate it. Dr. Fuster was already on it. He collaborated with Mount Sinai data scientists to publish findings—just weeks after the protocol was established—showing a strong relationship between use of anticoagulation drugs and improved survival from COVID. (You can read more about how big data informed anticoagulation treatment in Chapter 13.)

⚛

PRONING

'Then dramatically you see, whoosh, an increase in the air circulation'

"HE WAS COMPLETELY struggling to breathe." Jessica Montanaro, the Mount Sinai Morningside nurse, described a particular COVID patient in the ICU, one who was typical of many. He came into the hospital on a high-flow nasal cannula, a noninvasive breathing apparatus, and was quickly elevated to mechanical ventilation—to little avail. "His oxygen saturation was in the 70s—you really want someone to be at least in the 90s—and he was crashing," she said. "He was on one hundred percent of oxygen and other high settings on the ventilator. What do you do when someone's on one hundred percent of oxygen with an artificial airway? You don't have a lot of options."

So clinicians turned to a low-tech, high-touch intervention proven to help people with ARDS breathe a little easier: they turned him on his belly, a technique called proning. "It wasn't a planned thing," Ms. Montanaro said. "It was just, 'We have to do this, we have to do it now.'"

Immediately, his oxygen saturation levels rose, and clinicians had time to work to stabilize the patient. "You run out of things to do," said Ms. Montanaro. "So we did salvage therapies to try to at least mitigate things."

"PRONE VENTILATION has been around for a long time, and it has been shown to reduce mortality in ARDS patients," says Mount Sinai's expert in the field, Samuel Acquah, director of the Mount Sinai Hospital's medical ICU.

Normally in the ICU, ventilated patients are positioned on their back, in the supine position. That way, clinicians have better access to the patient, who is sedated and often on a paralytic, and to the critical equipment and medications.

But when breathing is in trouble despite the highest ventilator settings, the architecture of the lung suggests a solution. The lung is wider and fuller at its back than at its front, which has a smaller surface area. With a patient—and a lung—lying supine, fluid and inflammation build up in the back of the lung. When you turn the patient prone, that buildup shifts to the front of the lung, to the smaller surface area. That allows the back of the lung, with its greater surface area, to expand and take in more oxygen. This improves the lung's elastic and viscoelastic (viscous + elastic, like a memory foam mattress) properties, improves oxygenation, reduces inflammation and other organ dysfunction—and reduces mortality.

Before the pandemic, Dr. Acquah had regularly used a proprietary specialized bed for proning, a cage that secures the patient while the bed mechanically flips the body over. With a lung-involved pandemic on the horizon, Dr. Acquah reached out to the vendor to see if he could order more beds. But they were fast running out of stock. At the same time, the doctor envisioned an enormous spike in demand.

Typically, the Mount Sinai Hospital proned five to six patients a year.

At the peak of COVID, the hospital would go on to prone more than thirty patients *a day*.

"We recognized we had to go a different way," said Dr. Acquah.

That is, manual proning: a highly choreographed and labor-intensive process using six sets of hands to carefully turn a medically fragile ventilated patient from back to belly, minding the life-sustaining tubing. At first, Dr. Acquah and his team started training nurses, thinking they would be on hand in the units if proning was needed, and could form a team with physicians and respiratory therapists. But the need for proning grew exponentially—from two patients a day, to six the next day, to sixteen the day after that. And nurses were already overwhelmed with patient care.

That got cardiology nursing leaders Eileen Hughes and Dorothy Aguila thinking. With elective surgeries and labs closed, there was a corps of strong, skilled health care workers recently sidelined, including operating room and lab technicians. Could they be trained as a proning team? Over the course of forty-eight hours, with a combination of in-person and video training, they were. So, too, were staff redeployed from other shuttered units across other hospitals, including orthopedic surgeons, neurosurgeons, anesthesiologists, physician assistants, nurse practitioners, and physical and occupational therapists.

Here's how the proning teams worked:

First, the PPE. Full-body white hazmat suit with a gown over it (the hazmat suit protects the body; the gown protects the hazmat suit). N95 mask with another mask over that. Goggles, eye shields, gloves, shoe covers. "You can imagine, it was like a sauna," said Patrick Mullings, an OR tech at the Mount Sinai Hospital trained and redeployed to Mount Sinai Brooklyn's busy proning team.

Once assembled, with PPE donned and all necessary supplies in hand, the team entered the negative-pressure room. A respiratory therapist or certified registered nurse anesthetist was responsible for maintaining the airway. The rest of the team was posted bedside and ensured that the patient's many intravenous lines and catheters were visible and out of the way. Then, with a chuck—a bed underpad designed for moving patients—or a bedsheet, the team did the heavy lifting. "Make sure the Foley [catheter] and all the lines are up and nothing is compromised," said Mr. Mullings, who, before redeployment, positioned orthopedic spine patients for surgery. "Then we'll move them to the edge of the bed—that's the first lift. Then, making sure the a-line goes over the top of the patient, we would roll the patient to one side, tuck a sheet under them, then roll them to the other side."

With little room for error, team members all knew their stations at the bed and their role in the procedure. At Mount Sinai Queens, ICU nurse Geneline Barayuga joined redeployed physical therapists and physician assistants, as well as a respiratory therapist and wound care specialist, on the Mount Sinai Queens proning team. "We were able to meet before we started so that we know: you take care of the head part, you take care of the foot part, respiratory takes care of the intubation and making sure all the lines are free from being tangled and being pulled out," she said. "It was hard work. It was a team effort."

The teams were on constant rotation. Patients remained in the prone position for sixteen to eighteen hours, then needed to be returned just as carefully to the supine position. Mr. Mullings' team did up to twenty prones in a day. The team was stationed in the tiny lobby, where the security desk might be called to alert them to a mission. Or, if members of the team were elsewhere in the hospital, they would hear overhead, *Proning team needed, ICU three, bed four.* "It got very hectic very quickly," said Mr. Mullings.

Michael McCarry, head of perioperative services for the Mount Sinai Hospital, had been dispatched to Brooklyn to reorganize that overwhelmed hospital, and he quickly assembled redeployed surgical techs (including Mr. Mullings), central supply, and ancillary staff into the proning team. Mr. McCarry steadily got them the necessary equipment to make the laborious process more efficient, and he extolled the work they did. "This is an untold story that deserves to be talked about," Mr. McCarry said. "They sometimes washed the patients and changed their dressings as they turned them. It became almost a holy mission."

Clinicians determined the proning list by watching the so-called P/F ratio, the oxygen in the blood in relation to the setting on the ventilator. High amounts of oxygen coming from the ventilator and low oxygen in the blood spelled trouble—and the proning team would be called in to work its magic.

"You flip them over and within one or two hours you see a dramatic increase in their oxygenation. People go from, let's say 80, which is very borderline, all the way up to 180, 200 within an hour," said Dr. Acquah, referencing that P/F ratio. "It was a very dramatic response. The proning teams were very astonished and amazed."

So, too, were clinicians on the floor, stretched to—or beyond—their limits, caring for so many desperately ill patients. "To look at these patients who are at the brink of dying ..." said Dr. Acquah, setting the scene. "And then you called this team, who waltzes in and with their bare hands—it's not a medication—physically flips the patient over. You take somebody on the brink of losing their life, and then dramatically you see, whoosh, an increase in the air circulation. For everybody involved, it was a big break."

⁝

STANDARDIZING PROTOCOLS
'This worked for us. Take it.'

"HOW COULD ANYBODY be an expert?" asked Dr. Aberg. Honestly, if anyone could be, it would have been she. A well-known expert in HIV/AIDS, Dr. Aberg had built Mount Sinai's clinical trials unit, which was deployed throughout the pandemic to offer investigational therapeutics across the health system. She had been invited by Dr. Fauci to sit on the NIH COVID-19 Treatment Guidelines Panel and was at the center of many national and global conversations on pandemic strategy. "We've never seen the disease before, and we didn't know what to do. So there were no experts. I feel very confident saying I don't know because I don't. You had to be able to say that. We learned as we went along. Everybody shared knowledge. Everybody was in this together. Everybody wanted it to be better."

At Mount Sinai, clinicians and scientists were furiously consulting with one another and with colleagues around the country and around the world, sharing ideas and insights, papers, and protocols. Dr. Aberg, for one, studied guidelines from countries a few weeks ahead of the United States on the COVID curve—Italy, Spain, France—and shared her own findings and guidelines with colleagues in New York and in other cities weeks behind New York's curve, including Boston and Philadelphia.

Before Mount Sinai admitted its first patient, Dr. Powell had invited special guests to the weekly steering meeting of his division, pulmonary, critical care, and sleep medicine. Dr. Powell had had a longstanding academic collaboration with colleagues in Sichuan, China, who had flown to Wuhan to care for patients during the world's first wave of the novel coronavirus right at the start of 2020. Videoconferencing via WeChat on March 2, the Chinese colleagues told the Mount Sinai team about lessons learned, including, first and foremost, that personal protective equipment works. China had lost many care providers early on, Dr. Powell explained, but once they put strict PPE measures in place, the clinician deaths dropped markedly. The clinical takeaways included findings that Mount Sinai clinicians would soon observe themselves. COVID symptoms, the Chinese doctors said, seemed not only to be respiratory but also to include inflammation and blood clots. And treatments to consider—which Mount Sinai soon would—included steroids and anticoagulants, or blood-thinners.

"We had no real data yet from randomized controlled trials," said Dr. Aberg. "It was all from observation. It was based on hearing what others observed, as well as constantly mining our own database to try to understand how people respond: did we see any hint that a certain drug or a certain strategy may improve?"

This careful observation and close collaboration had led to the convalescent plasma program, the anticoagulation protocol, and the proning teams, all of which seemed to move the margins in patients' favor. On other fronts, clinicians quickly wrote and shared protocols to standardize new therapeutic interventions as well as traditional care made new by the exigencies of COVID-19. By codifying their early learnings, Mount Sinai clinicians ensured that all patients would receive the full benefit of hard-won advancements.

This extended to patients throughout the system, something that the chief medical officer of Mount Sinai's newest hospital on Long Island was acutely aware of. "We benefited in so many ways from being with the system and, specifically, clinically, with so many experts to help us with our protocols," said Adhi (Rob) Sharma. "We were not a standalone hospital trying to figure this out on our own, fumbling around the dark. We had the bright light of Sinai shining down on us, guiding us through this really tumultuous time."

Protocols out of Mount Sinai delineated a COVID treatment pathway based on disease staging—mild, moderate, severe, and critical, similar to how the NIH staged the illness—and outlined the care recommended at each stage. Continually updated and residing in the electronic medical record, this pathway gave care providers across Mount Sinai the first roadmap through a chaotic and rapidly changing landscape.

Mount Sinai's Institute for Critical Care Medicine drafted among its many guidelines (including a thirty-page *Handbook for Management of Critically Ill COVID-19 Patients*) a detailed protocol for a particularly fraught procedure, intubating during COVID. "It was not simply going into the room, taking your GlideScope and intubating a patient," said Dr. Roopa Kohli-Seth, director of the institute, which oversees critical care across the health system. "We had to go in there in full PPE and one hundred percent prepared—it's not that you could run out to go bring a medication."

The protocol thought of everything: "*Who will go in, who will be the first assist, what medications would go in and when? What would you wear? What equipment do you need?*" Dr. Kohli-Seth enumerated. "We protocolized all that. You will not go in without all this. And this person will be your first assist in the room, your second assist is outside the room. We had a backup plan, too. If the most competent person is busy intubating another patient, who is the second in command? Who's the third? Because there was a time, in the middle of the night, we were intubating six COVID patients at the same time."

MOUNT SINAI'S emergency room volume of COVID-19 patients went from a trickle to a steady stream to an overwhelming rush over two weeks in March, said Eric Legome, chair of emergency medicine at Mount Sinai West and Morningside. Somewhere between a trickle and a stream, he realized that the only way to get through it was to develop consistent guidelines and standardize care. Dr. Legome scrutinized the scant evidence from other hospitals ("if not best practice, based on any sort of real scientific evidence," he said, "at least what are other people doing?"), talked to a lot of people, and teamed up with Evan Leibner, an emergency medicine doctor at the Mount Sinai Hospital, to draft comprehensive guidelines. They offered a vivid window into the drama of Mount Sinai's emergency rooms. The protocol detailed how to navigate constantly changing testing practices, to understand the volatile progression of the illness when admitting or discharging, and to mitigate the dangers of performing CPR and intubation, aerosolizing procedures, on COVID patients.

Because patients were crashing and dying in emergency departments more quickly and in more exigent circumstances than ever before, the emergency department guidelines also addressed palliative care, including talking points to help families understand their next steps after a loved one's death in the cruel COVID era. "As you may know, because of the scale of the tragedy in this crisis, the traditional morgue may be at full capacity," clinicians found themselves having to tell families. "So we have increased our capabilities and capacity on site, in the form of mobile facilities. ... It is possible that the body of your loved one might be placed in one of these external mobile facilities. We are treating the deceased with the same integrity and care at all sites." ED workers also had to let families know, "Sadly, due to this crisis, funeral homes may be experiencing delays."

The first set of guidelines was published April 28 and would go on to be updated twelve to fourteen times in the next few months. Each time, protocols were shared in daily huddles, sent to attendings, the senior doctors on service, and flagged in the system's electronic medical records. In June, as the COVID census slowed down at Mount Sinai and ramped up elsewhere in the country, Drs. Leibner and Legome published the guidelines as a monograph in *Evidence-Based Medicine*, a peer-reviewed journal, so other ED clinicians could access them. "No one had any problems saying, 'This worked for us. Take it,'" said Dr. Legome. "We thought it was useful, and if anybody wants it, they should be able to use it."

There was a major caveat: Everything is fluid. "We were very clear saying, 'These are the guidelines as they are *today*,'" said Dr. Legome.

PART 2

THE GREAT MOBILIZATION

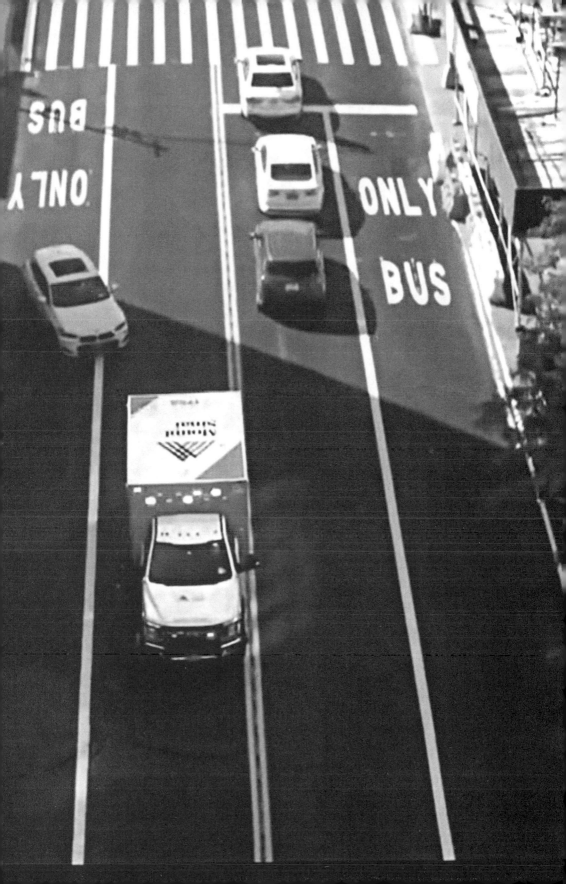

4 | THE POWER OF A HEALTH SYSTEM

*'The systems are really where the
magic happens'*

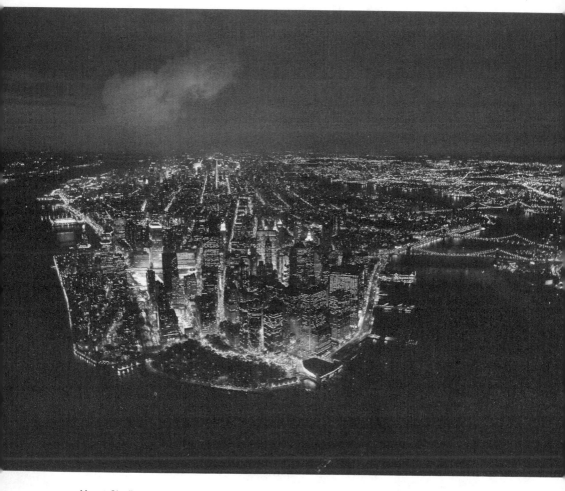

Mount Sinai's research-driven health system, spanning New York City and surrounding
communities, was the epicenter of the epicenter early in the pandemic.

AMID PERSONAL MEMORABILIA that Brendan Carr keeps from the brutal first pandemic wave is a photograph of his bedside table, which contained, as he saw it, the story of life at that moment. There was the family photo and two books salient to his new job, *MBA for Healthcare* and *A Theory of Justice*, the political philosopher John Rawls' disquisition on distributive justice. "This is as the whole country is talking about allocation of scarce resources and equity," noted Dr. Carr. There was also a draft of Dr. Carr's last will and testament, as he and his wife, also a physician, reevaluated their mortality, especially the question of who would raise their three children. Further to the idea of mortality, the nightstand also held a thermometer for daily requisite temperature-taking and a pulse oximeter to monitor blood oxygenation, just in case.

Brendan Carr had an awfully short on-ramp to his new job as the Mount Sinai Health System chair of emergency medicine. He started February 1, and Mount Sinai had its first COVID patient—the first in New York State—on February 29. Perhaps it was a blessing that it was a leap year, to give him an extra day on the job. A month later, the system would have more than 1,600 COVID patients. An emergency physician and health policy researcher whose work has focused on creating better systems for delivering more accessible emergency care, Dr. Carr had a background in academia as well as government, having worked in the U.S. Department of Health and Human Services seeking to improve trauma and emergency care services at the national level. That included work with the Departments of Veterans Affairs and of Defense to integrate military and civilian health care response during disasters and public health emergencies.

Dr. Carr views response to crises such as natural disasters and epidemics through the lens articulated by the medical anthropologist and public health expert Paul Farmer. To have the best chance of recovery, of saving lives and building back, attend to the Four S's: Systems, Space, Staff, and Stuff. "You're going to need somewhere to put people, the *space*, and you're going to need the *stuff* to take care of them," Dr. Carr explained. "Someone's got to know what they're doing—that's the *staff*. And then the *systems*—the systems are really where the magic happens."

COVID-19 presented remarkable challenges across all four of the S's. Rapidly needed was *space* to accommodate both an unprecedented volume of critically ill patients all requiring complex care at once and stringent infectious-disease protocols to contain the highly contagious virus. *Stuff*, too, was a story unto itself, beginning with well-documented PPE needs amid a global shortage to protect health care workers who were more vulnerable than ever before. Also in the *stuff* category, ventilators were in short supply and high demand, and making sure there were enough on hand and on the horizon tested the health care system's ingenuity, resourcefulness, and relationships.

Joseph Mathew, head of critical care at Mount Sinai West, described how he and so many of his colleagues were glued to the numbers: *How many patients on the floor? How many going home and coming in? How many ventilators are left? How many high-flow nasal cannulas? How many negative-pressure rooms, how many beds?* "Every day," he said, "we were constantly counting."

As for *staff*, the three-dimensional considerations were enormous. In a clinical care environment the likes of which had never been seen before, staff would have to learn on the fly, requirements and skillsets constantly evolving. And they would have to shift around like soldiers in battle, rushing in where needed. It was a giant mobilization effort, to get the right staff to the right patients at the right time—safely and with compassion for each health care worker's situation. In addition, there were medical students whose lives and learning had just been upended, and whose education was being rewritten in real time.

The operational logistics—*systems*—had to be big-picture, flexible, and at once responsive and anticipatory in order to manage the urgent needs and rapid changes around the spaces, stuff, and staff. Systems would be needed to assess and build out hundreds of negative-pressure rooms and other safe spaces inside and beyond hospitals. Systems would be needed to source and distribute an exponential increase in PPE amid fast-moving protocols and vanishing supply chains; to reimagine ventilators and leverage community and industry partnerships toward that end; to redeploy staff, keeping them safe while reinventing team structures to handle an unprecedented volume of critical patients. There would be systems to house and feed staff working all hours and, in many cases, avoiding their own homes for fear of exposing their families to the virus. There were systems needed to load-balance patients, to move them from completely overwhelmed hospitals to slightly less overwhelmed hospitals. And information technology systems would need to be freshly built or adapted to the new COVID normal, whether that involved making it possible for thousands of people to work and communicate remotely or adapting the electronic medical record to include such elements as new COVID protocols, care delivered inside a Central Park field hospital, and telehealth, which scaled up by 1,000 percent.

THE ENGINE POWERING all these systems was the Mount Sinai Health System itself. The seven-year-old research-driven health system yoked eight hospitals together under one name and, slowly over time, under one operational system. It was a gargantuan endeavor, and it was, by all accounts, nowhere near complete integration at the start of 2020. Eight hospitals in eight different communities throughout Manhattan, the boroughs, and Long Island. Some 42,000+ employees, 4.5 million annual patient visits. Coming together, but slowly.

The pandemic, as it did with so much else, accelerated a trend already in motion: forging a single entity out of the Mount Sinai Health System, in both overarching mission and on-the-ground operations, managing and distributing spaces, staff, and stuff, as well as balancing patients and disseminating scientific and clinical advancements.

"I believe the response to COVID built the Mount Sinai concept, a system that has really come together," said Don Boyce, vice president of emergency management for the health system. "It's hard to create a system of individual hospitals. But in the moment of need—when we really needed to move patients from one institution to another, when Mount Sinai Queens and Mount Sinai Brooklyn were hit extraordinarily hard—the other hospitals in the Mount Sinai system were creating additional space that their geographic layout allowed them to accommodate. Moving patients from one Mount Sinai location to another really enhanced the system's response."

In an ongoing effort to share lessons learned, Jeremy Boal, a central member of the health system's emergency management team, told the Radio Advisory podcast about the complexity of logistics for Mount Sinai—indeed, for any health care system that was facing, or sure to be facing in the near future, the wrath of this pandemic. "We were always working to track down more ventilators or trying to cut another deal to get protective gear. And staffing was incredibly challenging. Critical care staffing is typically at a very high ratio, and that expertise is incredibly unique," said Dr. Boal, who headed Mount Sinai's systemwide communication during the pandemic and strived for a Churchillian tone that reflected honesty above all, clarity of shared mission, and optimism rooted in a firm belief that the team at hand was up to the task before them. "There were an endless series of hurdles that we had to get over on a constant basis."

Dr. Boal vividly recalled a turning point in early March when it became startlingly clear just what Mount Sinai, indeed all heath care workers in New York, were up against, the profound weight on their shoulders. This was during one of the many phone calls between health care leaders and New York's Governor Cuomo. Said Dr. Boal:

> We're hustling and hustling and hustling to get ready, to stay ahead of this tsunami that is coming. Then we get on this call with the governor, and he basically says—I'm going to paraphrase, but I'll never forget this moment—he said, *Look, you know in Western movies when there's a small band of people. They've been fighting a much larger army, and they're cornered, waiting for reinforcements. Somebody rides up and says, 'There are no reinforcements coming.'* The governor said, *Today is that moment. We're on our own, and we're going to have to do our best.*

Such was the federal response to New York in early March. There were no ventilators coming from a federal stockpile, no army of health care workers or bundle of funds on the way.

That image, the dashed hopes of an embattled soldiery, alarmed Dr. Boal. But in the very next moment, the way forward became eminently clear: All in. Everyone. All the time. "It galvanized us even more to attack everything in real time," he said. "We're going to save every life we can save. We're going to take care of every last employee we can take care of. We're not going to be able to save everybody, but we can't stop. We can't slow down."

Attack everything in real time. Save every life possible. There was only one way to do that: working together.

‡

BECOMING A SYSTEM
'It was so beautiful to see our entire logistics switching'

ADAPT OR FALL BEHIND. Merge or submerge. Such was the health care landscape in 2013 when the Mount Sinai Medical Center—a well-known Manhattan hospital integrated with a highly ranked medical school—got together with Continuum Health Partners to create what would become the largest private health system in New York City. The goal was to bring Mount Sinai's standard of science-driven medicine within easy reach of all New Yorkers, and create an entity better positioned to weather and lead through seismic changes in health care.

The Affordable Care Act, which began its first open enrollment period in October 2013, was expected to transform how medicine was going to be practiced, delivered, and paid for. Traditional fee-for-service medicine, in which hospitals got reimbursed per procedure or interaction, would soon be eclipsed by value- and population-based medicine, in which hospitals seek to keep people healthier and receive payments largely tied to outcomes. More and more people were living with more and more chronic conditions—diabetes, hypertension, congestive heart failure. They needed ongoing care, but it was rarely in a hospital bed. At the same time, advancements in science and medicine, including in minimally invasive procedures, meant more interventions required shorter hospital stays than in the past, or no hospital stay at all. Health care was shifting its locus from inpatient to outpatient, its modality from acute to chronic. Health care organizations were seeking the so-called Triple Aim: to provide higher quality, lower cost care to more people—a threading of the needle that demanded greater economies of scale and would benefit from a larger patient population. Hence, mergers.

The Mount Sinai-Continuum merger was one of 98 hospital and health systems mergers or acquisitions that year. The Continuum hospitals, a citywide collection of freestanding hospitals with deep roots in their communities, would gain access to Mount Sinai's unique brand of medicine on the cutting edge of science. And Mount Sinai would expand its reach and expertise to more people. The thinking for both parties was that they would be better able to navigate rapid changes in health care together, to succeed at the business of medicine, to anticipate and master changing care delivery systems, and to deliver to more people the discoveries happening at the Icahn School of Medicine. They could consolidate the back-office expenses of the hospitals—human resources, IT, billing, compliance—in order to invest more in clinical services, develop centers of excellence, push the frontiers of medicine for the benefit of more people. In addition, the health system would begin to streamline certain services, consolidating and phasing out as necessary, with each hospital leaning into its areas of strength.

"The new Health System increases Mount Sinai's footprint from that of a local area to the entire island of Manhattan and beyond," Kenneth Davis, the health system's CEO, said in 2015, as the merger started to reify throughout the city, with hospital names beginning to change and strategies to align. "There is now a Mount Sinai doctor within walking distance of almost any community in Manhattan and within easy reach by public transportation of any neighborhood in the five boroughs and important suburban outposts. This means we are able to manage populations and position Mount Sinai for what the future of health care is going to look like."

Added medical school Dean Dennis Charney, "This is one of the very few places in the United States where a single top-flight medical school forms the foundation for outstanding clinical care across the full range of diseases, ethnic groups, cultures and languages, and socioeconomic class. When you're an institution like ours, where the hospital and the medical school are so intertwined and there is no university in between, you can focus wholly on health and making people well, on why patients come through our doors, why the ambulances are pulling up. Across the Health System, health and wellness, disease and its pathophysiology, diagnosis, treatment, and prevention stare you in the face every day."

When asked in 2021 whether anything like the capacious pandemic we were all living through was on his mind in 2013 as he negotiated what now feels like a prescient merger, Dr. Davis was quick to say, "Never. Never." But over the years—driven by clinical excellence, groundbreaking research, and an ever-shortening distance between the two—the Mount Sinai Health System had been growing into an organization that would reveal itself in 2020 to be broad-based, harmonious, and resilient enough to deliver the best care to the most people; to level-load space, stuff, and staff; and to lead through the largest health care crisis in modern times.

A HEALTH SYSTEM is at its aspirational best a complex amalgam of integrated parts—and people—working together across the continuum of care to manage population health in the most cost-effective way and with the best outcomes. The patient, ideally, is at the center of care and does not fall through the cracks when, say, moving from one level of care to another or one hospital in a system to another; needing electronic medical records transferred from one clinician to another; or benefiting from the advanced science-based care that academic medical centers can deliver to the many sites in their system.

Since it formed in 2013, the Mount Sinai Health System had taken many steps toward integration, including formally renaming its hospitals under the Mount Sinai banner. Roosevelt Hospital became Mount Sinai West, for example, and its sister hospital, formerly St. Luke's, became Mount Sinai Morningside. The system had been consolidating back office operations and streamlining certain clinical services to avoid duplication among nearby hospitals. Before the pandemic, Mount Sinai had launched a massive fundraising campaign—

the first as a health system—during which it spelled out a vision of its integrated future, from strategically building and transforming spaces across its campuses to investing in clinical and research programs that capitalize on and benefit Mount Sinai's enormous population reach.

Also, fortunately, Mount Sinai had recently begun to focus on how best to position the entire system—not just individual hospitals—to surmount crises. In 2018, Mount Sinai hired Mr. Boyce in the newly created role of systemwide vice president of emergency management. One of the first things his office did was conduct a systemwide mass casualty exercise, stressing operations with a number of "patients" arriving at Mount Sinai emergency rooms throughout the city. "If something's going to fail, it should do so on a day that's not an actual crisis," said Mr. Boyce, explicating the 101 of emergency preparedness. Mr. Boyce drew on his experience in both the private and public sectors, including as state director for emergency management in Massachusetts, as the Region 1 regional administrator at the Federal Emergency Management Agency (FEMA), and most recently as deputy assistant secretary for the U.S. Department of Health and Human Services Office of Emergency Management.

A key reveal from the mass disaster exercise: the health system needed a different superstructure to manage an emergency than the one then in place at the time of the exercise. On the hospital level, the Incident Management Team (IMT) structure worked well, dictating with precision who is in charge of what tasks, all under a single incident commander. But at the system level, Mr. Boyce believed, the overarching coordination would best be done with a larger, less hierarchical group supporting the individual hospitals' incident management teams. This Emergency Operations Center (EOC) design was similar to models used in city, state, and federal emergency management organizations to manage large-scale emergencies. The informal motto of the EOC concept is: "An unfamiliar place where uncomfortable officials gather to make unpopular decisions based on incomplete information allocating inadequate resources for unanticipated requirements in too little time."

When the major crisis hit for real, Mount Sinai's Emergency Operations Center was called into place. At first, everyone gathered in a single conference room, no masks, no social distancing, as knowledge about the virus and recommended protocols continued to evolve. One day, sitting face to face with a colleague, Margaret Pastuszko had a realization. "Wait a minute," thought Ms. Pastuszko, who is the president and chief operating officer of the health system. "We are using a standard emergency response to something that is so different. We have everybody in this central place when the enemy is the disease that we can't see."

Thus began a slow decentralization of the central command. The group spread across multiple floors at Mount Sinai's 42nd Street administrative headquarters. Locations were demarcated into zones, and each zone had its own hand-sanitizing station. Each time you moved between zones, you had to hand-sanitize and undergo a temperature check. Then, the inevitable happened: in early March, someone in the EOC tested positive for COVID.

"That was an aha moment for us, that this disease could wipe out our entire command structure," said Ms. Pastuszko, noting that the positive test triggered quarantining for those in the affected pod, or zone. "We flipped completely. We sent everybody back home or to their offices, and we ended up on Zoom."

BEFORE COVID, Mount Sinai's hospital and system leaders held a daily huddle at 9 o'clock every morning, a check-in on the basic status of operations at each site and clinical quality indicators. Hospital leaders would report in on their patient census, bed usage, ED volume, and any adverse events in the past twenty-four hours that their colleagues should know about. The health system was indeed coming together, strategizing as a system.

At the onset of COVID, the huddles grew much more urgent, high-stakes, and frequent. Three times a day, hospital and system leaders, as well as key members of the EOC such as infectious diseases, information technology, and human resources, gathered over Zoom to discuss the urgent issues of the day, and the days ahead. Hospitals reported on their COVID patient census and, as the pandemic rampaged on, on their multiplying needs, including supplies, staff, and patient transfers.

COVID-19 was not exactly an equal-opportunity attacker. Outerborough hospitals were slammed, at first without really knowing it— so their staff was decimated, too, from the outset, falling sick with COVID. As the health system increasingly mobilized on an integrated footing, it assessed need and allocated resources, human and otherwise, as equally as it could among hospitals.

⁂

TRANSFERRING PATIENTS, BALANCING RESOURCES
'Send us more patients, we'll help you'

AS A SYSTEM, Mount Sinai has a network in place to transfer patients among the hospitals, to get the patient to the right place at the right time for the right level of care. Normally, Mount Sinai's patient transfer center moves some thirty, thirty-five patients a day, on average, among system hospitals. That number rose to as high as seventy-five as the pandemic peaked. A patient transfer typically begins with a doctor calling 1-800-TO-SINAI. The transfer center then reaches out to see "who's accepting and who's sending," looks to match patient to bed, attends to accompanying paperwork, and sends the patient via ambulance to the waiting hospital. Collaboration, always essential to the process, was amplified greatly during COVID, and included case management, social work, nursing, and clinical teams to ensure the right treatment plan.

"It's always a challenge optimizing systemness," said Abe Warshaw, senior vice president of access services, which includes the transfer center. Individual hospitals are, understandably, focused on their own space and patient needs, he said.

The pandemic shifted not only the operations but the outlook. The inequity of supply and demand was stark, with the smaller community hospitals, Brooklyn and Queens, flooded with patients and suffering from a lack of space and staff. COVID patients on the whole were sicker, and more capriciously so, making the timing of transfers incredibly complicated at the same time as patients in COVID wards were staying in the hospital much longer than acutely ill patients traditionally did. Beds were not clearing, and patients in the ICU remained on ventilators for longer periods.

"During COVID, we really learned to become one big system and leverage the resource benefits that systemness offers," said Dr. Warshaw. "Everyone appreciated how hard it was for everyone else, and everyone wanted to be part of the solution for patients. Load balancing and getting the patient at the right time became Job One."

The systemness that would come to characterize Mount Sinai's COVID response was not without turbulence, particularly in the beginning, when the severity and scope of the pandemic were unfolding anew every day, every hour. The depth of despair at the community hospitals outside of Manhattan was not immediately apparent throughout the system. For a time, Cameron Hernandez, executive director of Mount Sinai Queens, felt that system leaders "weren't understanding what was actually happening here." By comparison with his Queens hospital, he believed the Manhattan hospitals felt "like luxury." "The fact that I cannot walk down a corridor without running into five stretchers is ridiculous," he said.

Similarly, Peter Shearer, chief medical officer at Mount Sinai Brooklyn, found it difficult to convey how dire the situation was— the sheer crush of patients and dearth of space and staff—simply with numbers. "On the daily phone calls, people like me or Cam were saying, 'Well, we could use some more help,'" said Dr. Shearer, who in short order became the only member of Mount Sinai Brooklyn's leadership not to fall ill with COVID. "As much as I could on a daily basis give numbers into the system and say it's really bad out here, I think it was only fully known to people who were here on the ground seeing it and hearing it. The system's multiple moving parts were trying to find their way into a well-oiled machine, but they weren't quite there yet."

Two milestones helped "oil" the machine, accelerating the system's ability to balance patients, staff, space, and stuff. On March 21,

Mount Sinai began redeploying legions of its health care workers whose existing jobs had halted due to COVID, whether they were frontline workers in non-COVID-facing fields or support staff no longer coming into the office. Secondly, on April 1, Mount Sinai opened its field hospital in Central Park, adding another 68 beds to the complex patient-transfer matrix.

For Dr. Shearer, having redeployed and traveling staff dispatched out to Kings Highway, Brooklyn, would go on to transform the overwhelmed hospital, where about one in five workers was out sick with COVID.

And at Mount Sinai Queens, while ambulances continued to deliver patients to the crowded ED, there was also a counterweight: "Now," said Dr. Hernandez, "there was ambulance after ambulance after ambulance to pick people up and take them to elsewhere."

Jonathan Nover, Queens' ED nursing senior director, recalled with the nostalgia of a Caribbean vacation the April day when charge nurse Melanie Droz intrepidly arranged for 50 patients to be transferred in a single morning. "You know that feeling on vacation when you first step off the plane, and you see the ocean and feel the breeze?" said Mr. Nover, forever grateful to Ms. Droz and her team. "That's what it felt like to see 50 patients transferred before noon. For the first time in six, seven weeks, the ED was at a number where you could actually take a breath. Like when you finally get to your resort and look at the water and you're like, 'All right, I'm on vacation now.' We celebrated."

The goal of any emergency department, after saving and stabilizing lives, is to get patients out of the emergency department and into the appropriate level of care, whether that's an inpatient unit, ICU, step-down unit, or discharge. The problem during the COVID-19 pandemic was that patients who had made their way to the emergency department were usually too sick for discharge, and, on the other side of it, beds in other units were not opening up fast enough. The problem was exacerbated because unless and until a patient's COVID status was known, he or she had to be alone in a room to prevent cross-contamination—and many of the inpatient rooms at Mount Sinai Queens were not designed to accommodate a single patient. That further delayed patient flow through rooms upstairs, putting even more pressure on the ED.

But the system stepped up. Normally, said Mr. Nover, there's something of a "push-pull" with a transfer, with one hospital working hard to "push" the patient elsewhere for more appropriate care, seeking another hospital to "pull" the patient in. "But during COVID, the system was pulling," he said. "They're calling us on our cell phones on our unit lines. '*Send us more patients, we'll help you.*' The support we got from other facilities, pulling, was unbelievable."

That was the objective, said Margaret Pastuszko: to be proactive rather than reactive, to see the needs of an overwhelmed, understaffed Mount Sinai Brooklyn, an overcrowded Mount Sinai Queens, or a rapidly filling Mount Sinai South Nassau and redistribute resources, staff, and patients accordingly. "We tried to learn early what was going down the pipe, so we could say, 'Wait a minute, Brooklyn, you're so busy that if you get more patients today, you're going to implode. So before that happens, scour the units, find us five patients that we can transfer to create capacity for you to take new ones,'" said Ms. Pastuszko, who was leading the system's emergency operations as one of the four-member Unified Command Group.

"We tried to move everything upstream, so we weren't just reacting to the six patients that they were getting in the ED right now. We were reacting to *knowing* that they're going to get those patients in the ED today and wanting to create the capacity for them to be able to take care of those patients. We knew at all times what was happening everywhere, and we were able, to the best of our abilities, to re-balance."

That went for resources, as well, for beds, ventilators, stylets to connect tubing, personal protective equipment. "It was so beautiful to see our entire logistics switching," said Ms. Pastuszko.

Take beds. Her office had designated a "bed czar" at the system level, to assess bed needs and demands and arrange delivery accordingly. Months earlier, the Mount Sinai Hospital had ordered some 80 beds to update an earlier model. "They never got those beds," said Ms. Pastuszko. "Instead, those beds were shifted to another hospital that needed them more."

If the team learned from 7 a.m. morning check-ins that a hospital had only three ventilators left and the weekend was coming, more ventilators were on the way to the hospital that day. Sometimes deliveries were made, via rented van, from the warehouse Mount Sinai built on the West Side at the outset of the pandemic. Other times, deliveries were made however and by whoever could get there the fastest. That included medical students bicycling to hospitals to help unload PPE and the head of supply chain driving out to hand-deliver medical equipment one night near midnight.

"We were all making deliveries," said Carlos Maceda, vice president of supply chain. One Friday at 10:30 p.m., Mount Sinai Queens was running out of intubation sets. Mr. Maceda located some at one of Mount Sinai's off-site locations on 85th Street in Manhattan and drove right over. He called Mount Sinai's real estate office to send someone to let him inside (remember, it was Friday night at 10:30), and he called a building administrator to walk him through where to find the equipment. As the night closed in on midnight, he drove the half hour out to Queens, so clinicians could connect struggling patients to ventilators.

"We became a system back in 2013," said Dr. Hernandez, referring to the signing of the Mount Sinai-Continuum merger. "But it wasn't until the pandemic that I really felt like we were a *system*."

So when Margaret Pastuszko and Jeremy Boal got a desperate call from Scott Lorin, president of Mount Sinai Brooklyn, who was in a hospital bed sick with COVID, Ms. Pastuszko was able to say, "Hold on. You're not alone."

HOW A SYSTEM SAVED A SMALL HOSPITAL

'We can do anything, because it's us'

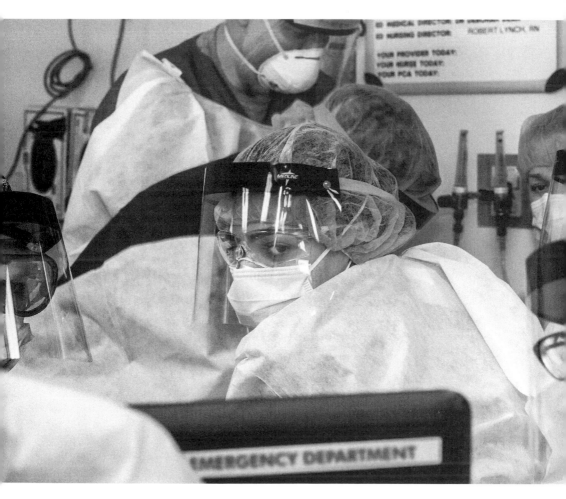

Mount Sinai Brooklyn's emergency department, with its 16 bays, cared for some 90 seriously ill patients at a time.

EARLY MARCH, 9:45 A.M., MIDWOOD, BROOKLYN—At the regularly scheduled bed board meeting to discuss the upcoming day at Mount Sinai Brooklyn, President Scott Lorin addressed the pandemic on the horizon. He pulled no punches, as Chief Nursing Officer Claudia Garcenot recalled: "He said, 'You guys, you can't imagine what it's going to be like. It's going to be bad.' And he said, 'People are going to get sick. We are going to get sick.' He said, 'People are going to die. Some people that we care about are going to die.'"

Like many of her colleagues, Ms. Garcenot could not yet wrap her mind around it. "I thought, 'Geez, you're being so pessimistic. Stop that. We're tougher than that.' I clearly remember thinking, 'That can't be. It's not going to be that bad.' And sure enough, in just a few weeks, it was."

⁜

IN THE BEGINNING
'It was the perfect storm'

PARKED ON EITHER SIDE of the three-story brick building was a pair of trucks that laid bare the life-and-death struggle inside this small hospital: a second oxygen tanker to help the throngs of COVID-19 patients breathe and two morgue trucks to handle, with as much dignity as possible, the hundreds who would not survive the deadly virus.

Mount Sinai Brooklyn, a former nursing home that evolved over the years into a hospital with many iterations of names, sits in the Midwood section across Kings Highway from a block-long yeshiva and across smaller side streets from tidy single-family homes and townhouses. The hospital serves diverse neighborhoods of Orthodox Jews, Blacks, Caribbean-Americans, and Russian immigrants. These were communities that, it turns out, were right in the line of fire. In the first U.S. wave, which swallowed New York and its environs, five out of the top twenty ZIP codes with the highest rates of COVID were in Mount Sinai Brooklyn's service area.

The hospital admitted its first known COVID-positive patient March 9. By March 16, the number of COVID admissions was doubling every two to three days, peaking in early April. Staff came to care for 50 percent more patients than the hospital routinely cared for; the emergency department cared for upward of 90 patients with only 16 bays. On April 1, there were 35 cardiac arrests or emergencies (compared with the usual two or three a day), 33 percent of patients required critical care, and 50 percent required respiratory support. Hence the additional oxygen tanker outside the hospital.

The first line of defense was the ED, ambulances streaming day and night to the humble emergency entrance. The higher acuity patients would be wheeled behind a plastic protective curtain and into the bustling ED itself. The movable walls between bays were all accordioned open, stretcher after stretcher after bed after stretcher packed together. The bays held more machinery and plugged directly into the hospital's store of oxygen, so that was where the more acute patients would go if they could fit, those on ventilators, high-flow nasal cannulas, BiPAP. In the middle of the room were the less-acute-but-still-acute patients who could be on portable oxygen.

Those who were even less acute could be treated just outside the emergency room, in the portable tent. It could house ten to twelve people at one time, sixty or seventy over the course of the day. The tent's grand opening in mid-March reflected the growingly familiar narrative arc of pandemic operations: it went up on a Friday during the surge with plans to open as needed, with staff training in the meantime. "As needed" became *right now*, and there was no "in the meantime." "We opened it Monday," said ED Nursing Director Robert (Bobby) Lynch. "We went live right then and there. There were no drills."

Mount Sinai Brooklyn's ED had become a massive bottleneck. Normally, Mr. Lynch explained, emergency clinicians stabilized patients and moved them upstairs. But now, patients were coming in at double the volume. And, with COVID patients, it was hard to tell when or if they were stabilized.

Secondly, space upstairs, in existing and newly converted ICUs, was not clearing out. COVID patients were, simply, not getting better.

They were remaining in their converted negative-pressure rooms, gravely ill, often on ventilators, for much longer without getting better than patients with other illnesses usually did.

Thirdly, the Brooklyn hospital was seriously understaffed, with so much of its health care workers out sick with COVID or quarantining with symptoms. That wreaked plenty of havoc on the flow of patients.

When the hospital asked to divert ambulances—something it doesn't like to do, but the small ED was bursting at the seams—the city declined. There was nowhere else to send people, no nearby hospital less overwhelmed.

"It was the perfect storm," said Mr. Lynch.

Among the life-and-death battles that emergency workers carried out day and night, ED Administrative Director Susanne Stefko recalled one small moment of heroism that captured the larger story of health care workers delivering compassionate, life-sustaining care any way and anywhere they could. It was the height of the surge, she recounted. There were no free stretchers and barely any free floor space. Stretchers were lined up bumper to bumper. Coughing, beeping, and a mechanical hissing filled the air. Rapid-response calls intoned overhead. Into this, a doctor who had himself become a patient needed treatment. The best that ED Medical Director Deborah Dean could do for him was to find a burgundy chair, an open space for it in the middle of the room, and a portable oxygen tank.

But that did the trick. Dr. Dean sat him down and was able to stabilize him. That image is seared in memory for Ms. Stefko as an example of how clinicians were able to make something out of essentially nothing. That was how this overburdened team in this overwhelmed place got through the earliest days of the pandemic and saved the lives it could.

AS MOUNT SINAI BROOKLYN went from bad to worse, over capacity with primarily COVID patients, gone were such clinical luxuries as checking on each ventilator three or four times in a shift, said Vadim Leyko, a respiratory therapist who remained in the hospital for days at a time during the peak, catching sleep where he could. "You just respond to emergencies, go from one room to another," he said. "And there were some instances when we responded to an emergency, and the patient was already pronounced [dead]. It was too late."

A respiratory therapist by training and a hospital administrator by dint of Mount Sinai Brooklyn's being a small hospital so everybody wore several hats, Mr. Leyko was also in charge of monitoring the hospital's oxygen usage. Emigrating from Belarus in high school, he had become interested in respiratory care from a book of medical professions he took out of the library. During the pandemic, he essentially became the oxygen guy.

COVID most often (though not always) manifested first as a respiratory disease, restricting the ability to breathe. On a macro level, the hospital itself mirrored the human struggle with oxygen. Normally, Mount Sinai Brooklyn is served by one external oxygen tanker, known as an oxygen farm. But after refueling demands proved too frequent, Mr. Leyko received another portable tanker, on wheels, which sat outside the hospital's emergency entrance, doubling the oxygen supply. The backup supply of portable oxygen cylinders was refilled every day rather than the usual once or twice a week, and went from an average of 70 cylinders on hand to 275.

"I've been here for sixteen years," said Mr. Leyko, "and in all our emergency preparations, I don't think we ever, ever discussed bringing in an additional oxygen farm because our existing farm wouldn't support the oxygen we needed in the building."

The oxygen farm was working so hard that its ventilator coils were icing over as they labored to convert the negative-300-degree liquid oxygen to a usable gas. The nimble, if overwhelmed, hospital quickly stationed someone next to the oxygen farm to pour hot water on the vaporizers almost around the clock, until employees could rig a solution: securing a hose over the vaporizers to keep a steady stream of hot water ensuring the flow of oxygen from tanker to lung.

IT WAS THE LAST FRIDAY in March. The 212-bed hospital was beyond capacity, mostly with COVID patients. Eleven patients would die that day, the most yet in a single day (although the hospital would go on to lose upward of eleven, twelve, thirteen patients a day for the next week). Scott Lorin had contracted COVID and was trying to run the hospital from a bed at the Mount Sinai Hospital. Claudia Garcenot, too, was seriously ill, and her twenty-five-year-old daughter would soon drive her to the same Manhattan emergency department. "I remember getting out of the car and not being able to hug her or kiss her goodbye," Ms. Garcenot said. "I just turned around and thought to myself, 'Is this the last time I'm going to see her?' Because I have never been that sick before."

Dr. Shearer, chief medical officer, was essentially, as a colleague described him, "a one-man show," as far as hospital leadership was concerned. Mr. Leyko had put in one stretch of some twenty-eight hours on his feet and had stopped going home entirely.

That's when Dr. Lorin, struggling to breathe between COVID and asthma, called Margaret Pastuszko and Jeremy Boal from his bed at the Mount Sinai Hospital and pleaded for help. "First of all," Dr. Lorin said, "I need to get leadership in there. Two, we need staff, and three, we need to transport patients out to hospitals within the system that are less affected, particularly Manhattan."

Ms. Pastuszko described the call as "the worst and the best in a single moment." As dire as the plea was to an already hard-pressed organization, she saw, too, the full potential of the Mount Sinai Health System—both that it was *Mount Sinai*, and that it was a *Health System*. "I thought, 'Okay, we can do anything, because it's *us*. It's not me, it's not him, it's not her. We care as much about the Mount Sinai Hospital as about Queens, as about Brooklyn, as about South Nassau. It's about *us*. It's about the team. It's about all of our employees.' I have to tell you, when Dr. Lorin said, 'We're imploding,' there was not an inkling of hesitation that our system would step up."

"Hold on," she told Dr. Lorin. "You are not alone."

Then she phoned Michael McCarry, a nurse by training and on the leadership team as head of perioperative services at the Mount Sinai Hospital. "We've got to go there," she told him. "He needs our help, our personal help." She knew that it was about more than just transferring patients and sending teams—although that was vital, and Mount Sinai would certainly go on to do that. It was now about getting boots on the ground in the devastated hospital, restoring leadership, and letting the exhausted staffers know "that we have their backs." She also hoped that an infusion of interim leadership would allow Dr. Lorin to sleep for a few hours as he battled COVID.

As the straight-talking Northern Irishman Mr. McCarry remembered it, Ms. Pastuszko began the call to him with, "Don't hate me for this," then she made her ask.

Answered Mr. McCarry, "I'll be there tomorrow morning."

÷

THE BENEFITS OF A SYSTEM
'It really felt like the cavalry'

SIX-THIRTY TOMORROW MORNING, to be exact. Mr. McCarry picked up his colleague Linda Valentino, the system's vice president of nursing, who would return to her old stomping grounds—she used to be CNO at Brooklyn—to co-lead the team with him. The two drove to Mount Sinai Brooklyn, a journey they would make every day for the next couple months. "Just about every corner of it was overwhelmed with COVID patients," Mr. McCarry said of his new hospital. "The ambulance sirens just kept coming and coming. The ED was packed. The scene in the emergency room was like something out of a war zone. A number of their staff were furloughed at home with COVID or suspicion of COVID. Everybody was just overwhelmed."

Opportunities to make change presented themselves from the moment he stepped in the front door. The current setup had health care workers enter the lobby, climb a few stairs to the right, snake down a narrow corridor, turn left down another corridor, and there, at the nursing office, was where they'd get their PPE. That's an awful lot of steps through a nearly COVID-endemic hospital without PPE, a lot of time for virus to gather, anxiety to build, fear to mount.

So, first things first. He and a team secured some wire carts and moved all the PPE to the lobby, so as soon as staff arrived in the morning, they secured the necessary equipment to do their day's work. It also became clear to Mr. McCarry that every staff member at the cramped, overrun hospital should be wearing an N95 mask. Health care providers working directly with COVID patients, of course, already were. But everyone, including people in housekeeping, pharmacy, and food services, should have the highest measure of protection available. In addition, everyone should have scrubs to change out of at the end of the day and leave, along with any contagion, safely stored for cleaning at the hospital. "Things were getting bizarre at one stage," Mr. McCarry said. He'd heard reports of people driving home naked, changing on the street outside the hospital, or stripping in their apartment hallways to keep the virus from coming home on their clothes.

While they were scarce and dear, Mount Sinai had on hand the N95s it needed to arm health care workers according to the infection-prevention guidelines of the day (which were changing by the minute, as national and local experts' understanding of the virus changed). But before he expanded the Brooklyn hospital's mask use, Mr. McCarry wanted to make sure his requirement would not threaten the system's overall supply. He wanted more than just a data point, more than just an email or telephone confirmation. He wanted to meet Carlos Maceda, head of supply chain, at Mount Sinai's warehouse on 110th Street and First Avenue. "I need to see what you have in reserve before I make that decision," Mr. McCarry told Mr. Maceda. "I don't want to do something that will deplete other areas of the system."

Mr. McCarry was comfortable with the reserve he saw, and the new mask policy went into effect immediately upon Mr. McCarry's return to the hospital. "When we were able to hand out those masks to every single staff member at the door of the hospital, and a pair of scrubs that they could leave at the hospital so they weren't bringing things back to their family, you could feel the relief in the air," he said.

Working hand in hand with infection prevention, Mr. McCarry and Ms. Valentino began outlining spaces in the red, yellow, and green tape that was becoming familiar across the system, designating COVID (red) and COVID-free (green) spaces, as well as transition zones (yellow) in between, to increase safety and minimize PPE usage.

With Mr. McCarry on site, the hospital could also more agilely connect to resources. When the emergency room ran low on stylets—a tiny but vital component of intubation—because clinicians were going through a month's supply in two days, the system made sure replenishment got delivered. "The system was constantly sending things we needed," said Ms. Garcenot. Even extra phone chargers, so isolated patients could call their families.

When Mr. Leyko reported that the hospital was low on ventilators, Mr. McCarry not only saw to it that dozens were delivered, but he also went the extra mile—indeed, the last mile—to make sure an overworked respiratory therapist could immediately *use* the machines. They arrived packed in boxes and, as it turned out, missing connective hoses. "Under normal circumstances I will have staff who will unpackage it and set it up and get it ready for use, but I didn't have anybody," said Mr. Leyko. "We were running from patient to patient every twenty minutes. You don't have time to breathe."

Exemplifying the importance of having leadership in place on the front lines in a pandemic, Mr. McCarry made a phone call, worked a little magic, and, "by morning," Mr. Leyko said, "I had the forty machines operational."

THE KEY TO THE TURNAROUND was when redeployed staff began to be dispatched out to Brooklyn—ultimately, almost 200 nurses and physicians from across the health system. Nurses from the New York Eye and Ear Infirmary helped out medical teams, plastic surgeons worked in the ICU. In addition, 90 temporary visiting staff—known as locums—came to Brooklyn from all over the country. They worked in new positions, outside comfort zones, at all hours of the day and night.

That included people like Dan Herron, chief of bariatric surgery at the Mount Sinai Hospital in Manhattan, who came to Mount Sinai Brooklyn and did whatever needed doing, whether that was transporting patients on gurneys down the hall, adjusting ventilators, or carrying out old oxygen tanks and bringing in new ones. "Everyone did everything," Dr. Herron told *New York* magazine, which published a series about the small hospital's response during the COVID surge in March and April. "It was heartwarming seeing everyone rising to the occasion and figure out what needed to be done and doing it. It's such an awful situation and yet it was also an extraordinary learning experience."

And that included people who could hit the ground running, for whom Peter Shearer was eternally grateful. "I had a fifty-five-year-old Staten Island cardiologist essentially staffing a unit like a medical intern, and very enthusiastically so, because he could identify patients who were improving, identify patients who were deteriorating, be a constant resource for nurses and their questions—which is something that we don't always have here in the hospital," said Dr. Shearer.

There were even enough nurses now to connect sick or dying patients with families, something that heretofore had been a luxury with a staff pressed to its limits. Said Ms. Garcenot, "We were now able to have redeployed nurses go from bed to bed or stretcher to stretcher and set up FaceTime calls between patients and their families."

From Mount Sinai hospitals and outside agencies, the emergency department received teams that each included a doctor, nurse, and medical assistant, Deborah Dean explained, gesturing to the entrance of a quieter ER many months later but as if she could see the mirage of them now, riding in to help with battle.

"It really was like the cavalry came," said Bobby Lynch.

Mr. McCarry fought hard to hold on to redeployed staff. Soon, the other hospitals across the system were seeing their COVID count increase, and some leaders wanted to re-redeploy staff. In a phone conversation, Mr. McCarry said, "Let's numerically define *busy*. I have two nurses for twenty-four patients in the ICU tonight. If you're that busy I understand. If you're not that busy"—he confessed to using "a little bit of an expletive" here—"I don't understand."

Turned out they were not quite that same level of busy. "They got it," he said. "That bought us another little bit of time till we got some more agency staff in as well."

That outside staff included certified registered nurse anesthetists

(CRNAs), a much-needed clinical force during a pandemic that steals breath. "They brought a very valuable skillset," said Dr. Shearer. "They would be here days and nights. They could help put people on ventilators. If a patient was on a ventilator on a unit that usually doesn't manage patients on ventilators, the nurses on those units have never worked with the machines or the strong sedative medications like propofol that you need to give. These nurse anesthetists, then, were there not just to help administer the medication but also to teach nurses on the fly what they needed to know."

Visiting CRNAs brought Vadim Leyko his first moment of hope during the pandemic. Early April. Sunrise. He had been at the hospital all night. Now, he was going to meet three new CRNAs reporting for duty at Mount Sinai Brooklyn's east-facing glass-fronted lobby. "The sun is coming up on that side, so it's very bright and warm that early in the morning," he recalled. "They walked in and just said, 'Hi, we're here, we're CRNAs.'"

In four hours, Mr. Leyko oriented the out-of-state travelers on the hospital's processes and equipment, an orientation that typically takes four weeks. And, for the first time in many days, he went home and slept in his own bed.

6 | BUILDING FOR THE SURGE

'We filled 104 ICU beds, and patients didn't stop coming'

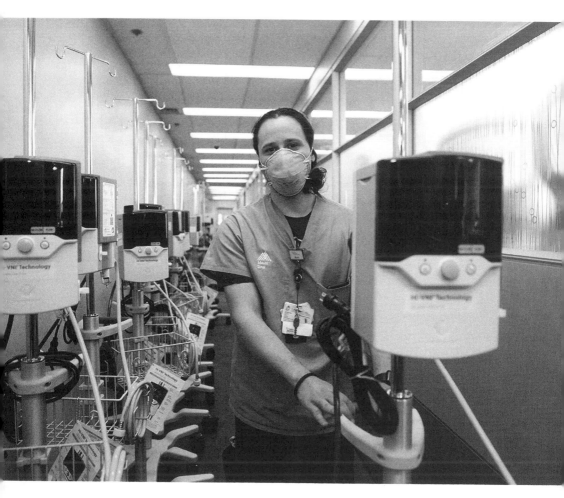

The Mount Sinai Hospital's respiratory care services went into overdrive to get much-needed ventilators to desperate patients. Above: Alvin Marin, equipment technician.

What are we likely to see in the next twenty-four hours? What is our plan so that we stay eight to ten beds ahead of the COVID patients? In the huddles, we would cover such things as the number of COVID patients currently in the emergency department, on the patient floors, in the intensive care units, awaiting test results. The numbers were increasing. We had to think, where are we going to go next? Which medical, surgical, and intensive care units were we going to surge into? Are we taking the transplant intensive care unit? Yes, we did that. Every day, we had to have a plan for the next unit to convert to an isolation/COVID unit.

—DAVID REICH, *president and COO of the Mount Sinai Hospital, outlining a typical discussion about its space as part of the daily huddle*

ONE OF THE VERY FIRST THINGS anyone knew about COVID-19 was that it was frighteningly contagious. As the COVID population surged across the Mount Sinai Health System, so too did the need to find—or create—tightly sealed negative-pressure spaces that would not exhale contaminated air into hospital corridors.

Dr. Reich was so immersed in the daily transformation of space at the Mount Sinai Hospital that he wrote a "Recipe for Creating a COVID Isolation Unit." After step 1, *Empowering Infection Prevention to lead*, step 2 was *Empty out a patient care unit*. In normal times, this would be almost impossible. But with Mount Sinai cancelling most nonemergency care and procedures, and New Yorkers avoiding hospitals for fear of the virus, many spaces throughout the hospital were already emptying out. So leaders of each of the eight hospitals could find rooms, units, and floors to surge into.

Step 3, *Physical preparation of the unit*, was the meat of Dr. Reich's recipe. This entailed vastly scaling up the health system's negative-pressure rooms by reconfiguring windows, doors, and airflow to create essentially a giant vacuum. "Engineers moved through the hospitals, in designated units replacing window panels in patient rooms with plywood," wrote Dr. Reich. "Each plywood panel had a large hole to accommodate the exhaust from a HEPA filtration unit placed in the room. ICU [spaces] without doors underwent construction to install temporary doors. All of this created negative-pressure rooms, preventing contaminated room air from flowing to the hallway while filtering and exhausting the contaminated air safely outside. Transportation removed most furniture other than patient beds."

Typically in hospitals, negative-pressure rooms are the province of infectious disease, which—until COVID—was a relatively small specialty and commanded relatively little space. There were 180 negative-pressure rooms throughout the Mount Sinai Health System, and they were not congregated together. Until now, an infectious disease had not swept through a New York population and demanded clinicians care for many infected patients in adjacent spaces, said Chris Hariegel, who led the effort as regional director of engineering for the health system.

But that was exactly what was needed now. Mr. Hariegel and his team went floor by floor, hospital by hospital, to mass-convert more than 500 medical and surgical rooms to negative-pressure rooms.

"Our engineering department could convert essentially any room with a window into a negative-pressure room," marveled Dr. Mathew, at Mount Sinai West, whose negative-pressure rooms could be spotted from the street. Look up as you walk across 58th Street, and you'd see a series of plywood windows, each with a telltale hose hole. Dr. Mathew sent pictures documenting the conversion to colleagues across the country, to help them prepare for what was coming their way. "Aside from the medical treatment itself, the capacity and the supplies to surge are very important," he noted.

Hard as the work was inside the rooms, it was equally challenging behind the scenes, said Mr. Hariegel. "As you can imagine, everybody was scrambling for the same equipment," he said, noting, too, that this was in a time of severe supply chain disruption. "There's only so many HEPA fans out there, only so many of the other pieces of equipment needed to convert these rooms."

In normal times, you can test for negative pressure by seeing if a piece of tissue gets sucked in under the door. For many reconverted COVID rooms, an informal test was much less subtle. Essentially, listen for the roar. Negative-pressure conversions varied from hospital to hospital, depending on the room configuration and the materials used. At Mount Sinai Queens, the resulting rooms—one in particular, an offline recovery unit converted to hold several beds and assistive-oxygen equipment—"sounded like you're in the engine of a jet," said Cameron Hernandez, the hospital's executive director. "You couldn't hear yourself think." But the rooms did their job: kept COVID from spreading through the building.

ON MARCH 23, with more than 20,000 confirmed COVID cases in New York and a steep rise still ahead, Governor Cuomo ordered all hospitals in the state to increase their inpatient capacity by 50 percent, and to double it if they could. Mount Sinai, which had 571 COVID patients at the time, including 109 in ICU, was already well on its way, reconfiguring spaces and adding new ones throughout the hospitals. Every bed mattered. Tents went up outside each hospital to alleviate burgeoning emergency rooms, among other purposes. Temporary patient rooms were beginning to be constructed in the soaring atrium lobby of the Mount Sinai Hospital campus, a light-infused space designed by I.M. Pei, more typically filled with the buzz and hum of medical students grabbing Starbucks before heading to class, heart patients checking in for appointments, physicians in lab coats or scrubs breaking from or en route to work.

Mount Sinai Beth Israel—the so-called "accordion hospital"—had been in the midst of shutting down its vast inpatient space when COVID hit. The square-block hospital on First Avenue had been ahead of its time in 1929 when it opened its doors with all private rooms, 500 of them. More recently, the hospital was positioning once again for a new chapter in health care, planning to greatly scale back inpatient care, move into a new 70-bed facility, and shift its focus to ambulatory care. Then came COVID, and Mount Sinai Beth Israel had something priceless: space. Pre-pandemic, the hospital maintained 24 critical care beds and 125 medical/surgical beds, with large sections of the hospital in the process of closing down. In March and April, the hospital tripled its critical care beds to 76 and more than doubled its medical/surgical beds to 308.

Uptown, at the Mount Sinai Hospital, critical care beds were rapidly filling up, and the hospital was about to do something that, in normal times, would seem heretical.

As director of the Institute for Critical Care Medicine, Roopa Kohli-Seth was responsible for ICU beds in the Mount Sinai Hospital, which, at the onset of the pandemic, numbered 104. "We filled 104 ICU beds, and patients didn't stop coming," she said. She and other hospital and critical care leaders brainstormed ideas. This one started as a blue-sky idea, a "silly idea," as Dr. Kohli-Seth recalled, but it began to gather steam: putting two patients in one ICU room. "Everybody said it cannot be done. I said, 'Let's try.'"

The equipment in an ICU—ventilators, pumps, monitors—and the volume of staff in and out to intensively care for a very sick patient usually make double-bedding prohibitive. But in its larger ICU rooms, the Mount Sinai Hospital simulated the scenario, two beds and two sets of life-saving equipment, and asked nurses, "Can you get around and still provide care?" When the answer was yes, Dr. Kohli-Seth said, "We are no longer going to simulate. We're going to put our first patients in there."

To Dr. Reich, that March 25 milestone marked a turning point. "The moment when we put two patients in an ICU room that was designed for one—and added another ventilator and patient monitor— that was very meaningful because it showed that we were not going to run out of space," he said.

PURPOSE-BUILT ICU ROOMS have glass doors, which was not always the case in retrofitted ICU rooms. Workers configured plexiglass windows or other see-through options where they could. But there were spaces where they couldn't.

How, then, to see behind a closed door?

At Mount Sinai Morningside, the infection prevention medical director, who was a new mother, had an idea. How about a baby monitor? A staff member dashed out to buy one from a nearby big-box store, and the team hooked it up. A step forward, but the images were quite small and could not cover both the patient and monitors. At the same time, Google, in conversation with Mount Sinai, wanted to donate its popular small, cyclops-eyed Nest home security cameras to help solve oversight issues.

"We were the first health system in the country to partner with them on this remote monitoring effort," said Robbie Freeman, a registered nurse who is vice president of clinical innovation. "The Google Nest is a consumer grade device—all you have to do is plug it in and stick it with a magnet to the whiteboard in the patient room." His team worked with engineers to connect the cameras to a console so clinicians could see many patients at a time. A nursing assistant watched the console continuously, keeping a special eye on at-risk patients and flagging patients who raised concern. Through the first wave, 200 Google Nest cameras connected patients and clinicians across Mount Sinai's hospitals.

✣

BUILDING A FIELD HOSPITAL IN CENTRAL PARK
'Mountains were moved'

Union first—peace next. And War last.
—SERGEANT EGBERT MCLAUGHLIN, *a Union soldier and patient in the Central Park Hospital, writing in 1864, the last time a field hospital was erected in Central Park*

IT WAS FRIDAY NIGHT, March 27, when Don Boyce called his colleague Brendan Carr. The two were friends from their previous work at the Department of Health and Human Services, and they were about to embark on a project that might have felt like it was straight out of those public-sector days. "What are you doing tomorrow at 8:00 a.m.?" Mr. Boyce asked Dr. Carr.

The answer was, as it turned out, meeting with representatives from the international relief agency Samaritan's Purse, who had just flown in from their base of operations in North Carolina and with whom Mr. Boyce had worked years before. After convening at Mount

Sinai's 42nd Street offices and discussing the relief agency's capabilities providing stuff and staff for a field hospital, the two organizations quickly made an agreement.

The rest of the Samaritan's Purse team, which had a field hospital packed in trucks and ready to go, then spent the day driving the six-hundred-plus miles from North Carolina, while the Mount Sinai team scouted the city for the right location for the tents that would help them care for patients beyond their overflowing hospitals. They decided on the East Meadow of Central Park, directly across Fifth Avenue from the Mount Sinai Hospital, for its combination of open space and proximity.

"They are self-contained," Dr. Carr said of the relief agency, "but it would be helpful if they could dip into the hospital's resources if needed. If their pharmacy could be back-filled by our pharmacy, if their supply chain could be augmented by our supply chain. They had all their own stuff, but sooner or later you run out of stuff."

Building a field hospital in New York City's crown jewel over the course of a single weekend required innumerable phone calls with many city agencies amid much goodwill. "They needed electricity, they needed water, they needed permits to do construction in a place that is like saying, 'Hey, do you mind if we build this on the Capitol grounds, or in the Sistine Chapel?'" said Dr. Carr. "That's what the East Meadow is to the Upper East Side. First time since the Civil War. The city was actually kind of amazing."

The field hospital went up quickly, crews jogging at times through a rising mist to unload equipment, roll out tarps, and site and inflate a series of white tents in the span of forty-eight hours. The field hospital was similar to the ones the relief agency had built in hot spots around the world, including an identical COVID hospital in Italy just two weeks previous—but was the first of its kind on U.S. soil. It would provide the space and staff to care for 68 patients at a time, including 10 in ICU beds.

Con Edison came out on Sunday afternoon and dug a trench across Fifth Avenue to convey electrical power into Central Park, so the field hospital did not have to run on a generator. The Fire Department of

New York stopped by to see where they could help. Mount Sinai's IT team erected antennas on the Mount Sinai Hospital to make sure the signal would get to the park, a system for oxygen was installed, and the field hospital was connected to Mount Sinai's electronic medical records. Much of the work, including Con Edison's labor and power, was donated to the cause.

"Just the involvement of everyone to make this happen—it's impressive to see what can be done when everyone puts aside everything else and knows what the end goal is and what can be done," said Mr. Hariegel. "Mountains were moved in a span of about three to four days, and we had patients in that week."

On April 1, the field hospital opened to patients. It treated 189 patients before closing shop a month later.

ALMOST AS SOON AS tents started going up, so, too, did controversy. Medical students and health care staff who had been volunteering to help set up tents discovered that the relief agency, an evangelical Christian organization led by the Rev. Franklin Graham, had an anti-LGBTQ stance. That flew in the face of the progressive values held by many at Mount Sinai, especially the students.

Their protest put Mount Sinai leadership in a difficult position. At the fulcrum point was David Reich, president of the Mount Sinai Hospital, who was completely attuned to his hospital's ever-growing need for more beds and patient care, and who was an openly gay man instrumental in a number of advances on that front, including Mount Sinai's groundbreaking Center for Transgender Medicine and Surgery.

"*David, it's my job to walk you over and introduce you to the leadership of Samaritan's Purse,*" Dr. Carr recalled saying as he rounded up Dr. Reich for the short walk across Fifth Avenue. Dr. Carr acknowledged the emerging controversy and apologized if the project had created a problem. "David said, 'Maybe I'm wrong here, but my understanding is that they're here to save the lives of New Yorkers. Nothing to apologize for, let's go say hello.'"

Dr. Reich does not relish retelling the story. But his position—both at the time and months later—was clear. "It's very challenging for me because I've dealt with decades of anti-LGBTQ sentiment," he said in an interview in September. "But in the circumstance, I feel that working with this organization was absolutely the right thing to do."

Together with medical school Dean Dennis Charney, Dr. Reich wrote an email to Mount Sinai's tens of thousands of employees, acknowledging the debate while embracing the partnership. "This virus kills people of every religious belief, ethnicity, gender identity, and sexual orientation," the two men wrote. "New York has lost more than 1,000 people already, and more are dying every day. Mount Sinai and Samaritan's Purse are unified in our mission to provide the same world-class care to anyone and everyone who needs it, no questions asked. We are all focused on one thing: saving lives."

☦

CONNECTING TO CARE AT HOME
'It found its place'

BEFORE COVID kept people out of the hospital for regular care, telehealth—connecting to a clinician by phone or video—represented a small fraction of care, maybe 25 such visits a day. Then the pandemic hit. Hospitals were overwhelmed with COVID care, and in- and outpatient facilities in the city largely closed to nonemergency care. Even with serious illness, patients avoided hospitals because they did not want to become exposed to the virus.

At Mount Sinai, innovation and information technology teams sprang into action, building out the infrastructure and buying hundreds of iPads amid crippled global supply chains, as an option for providers delivering telehealth (they could also use their own devices, via the Epic mobile app). Staffers even ran out to B&H Photo and Video and other local stores and bought up what they could. The health system went from conducting some 25 telehealth visits a day, a real outlier when it came to care delivery, to conducting the bulk of regular care this way: 5,000 telehealth visits a day.

"We increased our telehealth volume two hundredfold in the span of less than a week," said Paul Francaviglia, who headed the telehealth transformation as senior director of information technology. "The system development, the licensing, the standing up of support processes, the quick drafting of quick guides for people on how to use the tool—all of that really had to be done in an unprecedented timeline."

Early on in the pandemic, federal and state governments moved to expand access to and reimbursement for telehealth services, recognizing that this alternative care modality had suddenly become a core part of how Americans would be visiting with their clinicians.

"A year ago telehealth was a solution looking for a problem to solve," said Bruce Darrow, a cardiologist who is the health system's chief medical information officer. "It wasn't necessarily better, patients didn't necessarily want it more, doctors certainly weren't trained to do it, you couldn't make money on it, it wasn't reimbursable. You couldn't use it to talk to somebody across the bridge in Secaucus because you didn't have a license in New Jersey. As the barriers to being able to use it went away and the reasons to use it went up simultaneously, it found its place."

The former "solution without a problem" was now solving all kinds of problems. In addition to connecting patients at home with their clinicians, it was also used as a "forward triage system," as Dr. Carr called it—akin to the triage you'd find in an emergency room, with a clinician deciding who goes first, who needs care most urgently, who can be helped, who has a non-survivable injury. During the pandemic, there was another kind of triage system to determine which COVID or COVID-suspect patients should come to the hospital and who should stay home. "You call our telemedicine platform, and say, 'I don't feel well. What do I do?'" Dr. Carr explained, and the clinician on the other end would determine the best next steps. After all, the mayor and governor had issued stay-at-home orders. And hospitals were telling patients that if they were not short of breath, they should stay home. But people were afraid, and the illness could be volatile. "It was a super complicated time."

Even in the corporeal setting of the emergency rooms, triage was sometimes done virtually, with patients going into cubicles and meeting with clinicians via iPad. "So I don't have to go into the room and breathe your air" before clinicians knew what they were dealing with, explained Dr. Carr. Instead, the clinician determined next steps virtually: whether and where to admit.

Inside the hospitals, nurses also communicated to patients using an iPad—one inside the room, one just outside of it—to limit comings and goings from an infectious room. A new in-person kind of telemedicine for the COVID era.

ALL HANDS ON DECK

'There is no night, there is no day in COVID'

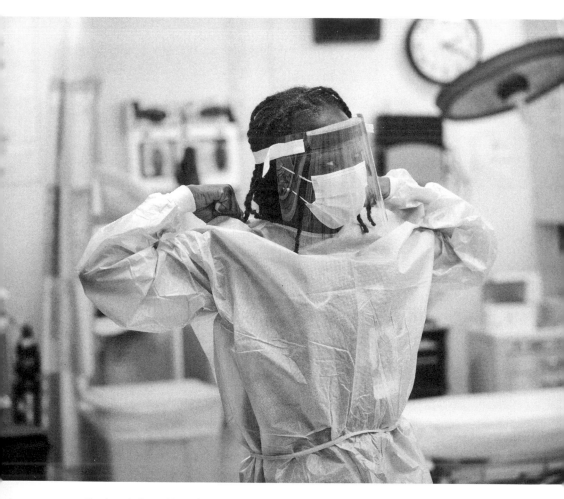

Kaedrea Jackson, Mount Sinai Morningside emergency physician, says her three young children "have noticed mom's not home much. But that's what's needed right now."

IN THE FIRST WEEK OF MARCH—with just a handful of COVID patients in Mount Sinai hospitals—Barbara Murphy predicted the unthinkable: that within three weeks, Mount Sinai would be caring for more than 700 COVID patients struggling to stay alive.

She was right.

"Based on the current volume and the doubling, I projected 760 patients with COVID within three weeks," she said in an interview months later, reflecting in her brisk Dublin accent on the literally incredible numbers during the first wave of the pandemic. "People didn't believe me, but we were bang-on with the numbers."

Before the patient census climbed that high, as patients started flooding into Mount Sinai hospitals across the city, Dr. Murphy knew the great urgency was to mobilize staff. On March 23, with 571 patients in the Mount Sinai Health System and nearly 100 new patients coming in every day, Dr. Murphy, chair of the department of medicine, wrote a simple plea in the contemporaneous notes she was keeping: *manpower manpower manpower*

SHE WAS GETTING frantic calls from Mount Sinai hospitals across the city, especially hard-hit Mount Sinai Brooklyn, requesting more staff. *We need people*, they were saying. *I need five teams, X number of residents, this, that, and the other.*

"This can't be 1-800-GO-BARBARA," she told herself. "We have to have a system in place to understand the needs and be proactive advisors." She, along with Marc Napp and key leaders across the department of medicine, reorganized the structure of inpatient care to cope with the overwhelming number of ill patients. Certain departments were more suited to sending clinicians to the ICU, she knew, and certain others were more suited to providing care elsewhere.

With elective surgeries and most other nonemergency care postponed, thousands of clinicians were ready—and eager—to be redeployed to fast-proliferating COVID units. A few days earlier, Dr. Boal had sent out a note to health system leaders describing the all-hands-on-deck call that was to be issued on March 21—asking staff to "register for COVID-19 duty." Dr. Boal likened this fight-of-a-lifetime to the war effort. He wrote:

> There is important work for everyone. We will be standing up a
> series of corps. In World War II it would have been things like
> ambulance drivers, machinists, and the like. For us, it will be
> everything from runners who can help carry equipment and
> supplies where they are needed, to scribes who can make it easier
> for our nurses and doctors to do their work, to people who have
> training in therapeutic support to care for our own traumatized
> staff, to specialized teams that can support the care of ventilated
> patients. There are so many ways to contribute, and we will need
> everyone in this fight.

By the end of the first wave, Mount Sinai would go on to arrange
1,641 staff redeployments. In addition, 758 outside temp workers filled
in in the COVID effort. Carefully constructed teams were deployed
around the clock. "There is no night, there is no day in COVID," said
Dr. Murphy. "Patients are the same at night as they are in the day."

Teams were restructured to better match the overwhelming need
in a certain few COVID-related areas—critical and pulmonary care,
for instance—with the highly diverse skills of the workforce at hand.
And flexibility was the order of the day, along with a generosity
of spirit needed to plunge into wholly new roles amid the fear and
uncertainty of the pandemic. The "staff" story extended well beyond
the workplace. COVID was not only a fight taking place in the hospitals, after all; it lived at home, too.

"The ability to change so rapidly into a completely different system
was absolutely phenomenal," said Dr. Murphy. "The management,
the oversight, the flexibility, the way they pivoted toward the crisis,
was really amazing to watch. There was a sense of purpose. People
realized this was a phenomenal crisis, and we have to step up and
work together and get it done. It was really tremendous if it wasn't
so awful."

Dr. Reich sketched the scene of Mount Sinai's deployment in an
April 17 presentation for a CDC clinician outreach and communication activity (COCA) call on insights from hospitals in the midst of
the surge. "We have neonatologists, pediatric cardiologists, orthopedic surgeons, rehabilitation medicine physicians, and advanced

practice providers that are now working with hospitalist teams and critical care teams," said Dr. Reich. "Everyone lost their original title and became something new. We put out educational materials about the management of respiratory failure and critical care of these patients. And the team-based care model means that everyone forgot about what their original role was and figured out what their new role was. And I have to say, people were very innovative and thoughtful about it."

Hundreds of physician assistants (PAs) were redeployed to support the front lines, leaving their home departments to care for patients in surge tents and COVID wards throughout the system. Orthopedic and neurosurgery PAs were redeployed to emergency rooms and tents, working outside their scope to help nurses draw labs and put in IVs. "I applaud them for stepping up to the task and doing a fantastic job," said Allison Chang, a PA at Mount Sinai Morningside and Mount Sinai West. "Makes me proud to be a PA."

MICHAEL MARIN OVERSEES Mount Sinai's department of surgery, with one hundred thirty full-time surgeons supported by a staff of more than five hundred. Nurses, medical assistants, PAs, billers, administrative assistants. In the middle of March, Mount Sinai cancelled all elective and nonemergency surgeries.

"Overnight, we were a different group of people," said Dr. Marin.

The next day, he sat down and created a redeployment plan for his department. Following the pandemonium of the great 2003 blackout that paralyzed New York City, Dr. Marin had created a platoon model of disaster staffing that would give everyone a role and best match staff to need. For COVID, he would divide his entire department into platoons, highly structured teams, and ship them out where and when they were needed. Specialty teams of surgeons were also dispatched across the system to help with skilled procedures that became unprecedentedly common during COVID, providing vascular access, performing procedures to allow for dialysis, and creating tracheostomies in patients in respiratory failure. The surgery vice chair, Paige McMillian, pivoted from managing the department's administrative and finance operations to configuring and maintaining a large command grid for the redeployment.

"We would get called: 'There's a disaster going on over at Mount Sinai Brooklyn in the ED,' or, 'There's a disaster at the Mount Sinai Queens ICU,'" Dr. Marin explained, noting that each platoon traveled with their own pre-packed PPE in a black Nike backpack. "And we'd deploy two to three platoons, depending on the size of the problem, rotating them to prevent fatigue. And they'd cover all day and all night."

The military precision at the heart of Dr. Marin's approach to redeployment was in part to manage the multivariable complexity of dispatching so many people to so many places under urgent conditions. And it was in part to combat the anxiety of the unknown, which was a defining feature of the times.

"We didn't just have a pandemic, but we had a pandemic where the pathogen was unknown, how to treat it was unknown, how dangerous it was was unknown, how it was transmitted was unknown," Dr. Marin said. "And when all this is unknown, people's imagination goes to their greatest fear. In my view of the world, the best way to fight fear is with organization."

Anthony J. Vine, a laparoscopic surgeon at the Mount Sinai Hospital, embraced his redeployment to Mount Sinai Brooklyn. As Dr. Vine wrote in a moving frontline essay in *The American Surgeon,* he was inspired when Dr. Marin told the team, "This is like nothing we've ever encountered. ... For now, we are no longer surgeons, nurse practitioners, residents—we all are equal healthcare soldiers."

Coming back home after his first day, Dr. Vine wrote, "I felt like I had returned from a foreign battleground, even though Brooklyn is just over the East River. ... Despite the fact that all ERs and ICUs essentially look the same, COVID caused so much human suffering that I was disoriented, as if I were in an unfamiliar land."

At Mount Sinai Queens, redeployed surgeons took on tasks that didn't necessarily draw upon their surgical skills but were equally life saving, said Cameron Hernandez. He recalled a day right near the peak, April 9, when the emergency room admitted 70—"seven-oh," he emphasized, so no one mistook it for 17—patients, who then waited for beds in the hospital. The patient count far exceeded the number of oxygen hookups in the wall, so dozens of patients relied on oxygen tanks to breathe. Dr. Hernandez knew where the redeployed surgeons could do the most good: "I needed two surgeons to literally go around the emergency room and check every tank," he said. "Just keep walking around, because if one of these tanks runs out, the person dies. I know they're surgeons, and they can assess while they're doing it— but I need a body to check each tank."

No questions asked. "People did it," said Dr. Hernandez. "There was no hierarchy."

Doctors in outpatient practices heeded the call, too, volunteering for redeployment on COVID wards. Long Island cardiologist Jay Dubowsky left his "comfortable clinical practice" for Mount Sinai South Nassau. He had trained in the time of AIDS at a New York City hospital and practiced during the racially charged 1991 riots in Crown Heights, Brooklyn; the World Trade Center bombing; and, devastatingly, 9/11. "And then came COVID," he blogged. "Treating COVID-19 patients created challenges I had never imagined. And it created opportunities I never considered."

At first, he felt out of his element, but the intensity of and commitment to the work at hand bound him together with his new colleagues, many, like him, redeployed from comfortable clinical practices. "We bonded over patient care. We bonded over the families who were unable to see their ill loved ones. We became the patients' families. We held their hands, stroked their heads, and held iPad tablets so the families could see their loved ones. We celebrated patient successes, their triumphant extubations, and their long-anticipated discharges. And we mourned their deaths, as one of our own. We all came together as a Mount Sinai family."

The city's hardest-hit hospital was Elmhurst, a public hospital with which Mount Sinai has a partnership, including sending classes of medical residents there to train. Arvind Badhey began his first day as chief resident of otolaryngology (or ENT—ear, nose, and throat) at Elmhurst on March 15. Elmhurst, like Mount Sinai, had canceled nonemergency surgeries, and Dr. Badhey and a team of eight to eleven residents joined the newly formed ENT-run COVID-19 unit. "I know more about intensive care than ever before and know how to better manage these critically ill patients," said Dr. Badhey. "We are swift critical decision-makers and more prepared for our future than we could have ever imagined."

His colleague Benny Laitman described entering the ENT-run unit of the hospital on one of the most fatal days of the pandemic in New York City. "Alarms were blaring, including the hospital oxygen alarms, as the room was not made to deliver that much O_2 at once," Dr. Laitman wrote in a blog, *ENT in the Time of COVID*, which he kept about the experience. "I was sweating profusely through my multiple layers of masks and protective gear. I couldn't hear a thing. We are outside of our comfort zone, managing critically ill and sometimes actively dying patients. But we are here, and that's what counts."

✢

REIMAGINING TEAMS

'The residents are really soldiers'

CLINICAL TEAMS WERE structured based not on seniority or title but on proximity to the knowledge needed to treat this infectious emergent illness. Often, it was the newer team member, the one with the fewest years out of medical school—the medical resident—who was in charge.

"If you were an orthopedic attending," Dr. Murphy explained, using the term for the senior member of the clinical team, whether an attending physician or attending surgeon, "you weren't an attending on one of our services. You were an intern, and it could be a chief resident or a senior resident that was now telling you what to do. Our residents have more experience with a critically ill patient than the attending or an orthopedic attending. You can't leave people out of their scope because it's not fair to them, and it's not fair to the patient."

The same was true on the surgery platoons. "The surgical residents were the ones most facile with moving around these hospitals," said Dr. Marin. "They do it all day and all night. The attending surgeons come in, they do their operation, but they don't know where's a lab cart, how to get things done. The residents are really soldiers who understood the infrastructure of our hospitals. So they led the platoon."

Teams were also organized by geography. Rather than having clinicians or teams be assigned to patients throughout the hospital, teams worked together and covered an adjacent cohort of rooms. If an average team covered 12 patients, the first team would be assigned to Rooms 1-12, the second to Rooms 13-24, and so on. That not only cut down on time spent moving from room to room—now a luxury on a floor where patients were coding much more frequently and decompensating much more vertiginously. In addition, because each team was covering a single finite space, the health system's infection prevention specialists approved a protocol to remain in the same PPE as they went in and out of rooms, conserving precious PPE and minimizing any risk that comes with continual donning and doffing. "All they had to do was change their gloves," said Dr. Murphy.

In fact, the Mount Sinai department of medicine wrote the primer on how to create teams during a pandemic surge. "Redeployment was a massive undertaking for our institution and may quickly become necessary for other health systems in the coming weeks as Covid-19 cases rise nationally and globally, or during future crises," the team wrote in *NEJM Catalyst* on May 4. The paper detailed "six overarching principles: (1) create an organizational structure, (2) define your need, (3) identify and optimize your pool of health care providers, (4) create surge teams, (5) prepare and deliver orientation materials, and (6) optimize working conditions for staff."

The primer both enumerates best-in-class operations and never loses sight of the visceral humanity at stake. In one striking detail: "While we did our best to anticipate learning gaps in advance, during the first night of deployment, a non–internal medicine PA needed to pronounce a patient's death, a task she had not performed previously. Subsequently, we incorporated 'how to manage a patient death' information into our onboarding learning."

THE LEARNING CURVE for the redeployed was steep. For those working on the clinical front, they had to learn not only a new team and a new place, they also, of course, had to learn how to care for patients with an infectious virus new to humankind and with no known treatment. "Because nobody knew what COVID was," said Dr. Murphy, "and there were no primers, we would say, *Here are the main things the patients have*—we didn't even really know at the time—*and here are the things that you should know.*"

It had been some twenty years since Joseph Herrera, a physiatrist, had studied critical care, and he'd never practiced it. So when he converted his Mount Sinai Hospital rehab unit into a COVID unit, he hit the books. "We received a lot of literature from our medicine teams," he said, noting that one in particular stood out. *"The Guide to Critical Care for the Noncritical Care Provider.* I spent nights, weekends, reading up, trying to get caught up on all the things that I knew in medical school."

Quickly, he found that there was one thing he was doing frequently, and something he had never needed to do as a physiatrist: resuscitating people who had stopped breathing. Although he had recertified his ACLS (advanced cardiac life support) every year, he was now treating more people who had stopped breathing in one hour than he had over the course of his career.

He shared his learnings with his Association of Academic Physiatrists colleagues in an April 23 email, from suggestions on how to structure teams and get through challenging days to the importance of getting back to basics: "I can't speak for everybody, but I was anxious about my own medical knowledge regarding the medical management of the critically ill patient and vents. I visited all of the recommended sites and read all of the recommended protocols. The most important thing that you need to know is ACLS. During my time on the unit, I started a number of codes until our code team arrived. I was even doing chest compressions. Know your ACLS."

Nurses also needed critical care training, and fast, to redeploy from a variety of specialties to where they were now needed most. Mount Sinai partnered with Sana Labs to develop Project Florence, a personalized learning platform to assess and enhance nurses' critical care skills and knowledge, using AI to detect competency gaps and create an online curriculum accordingly. Once developed, the platform was shared globally. More than 500 Mount Sinai nurses had trained on the program as of June 30, 2020, as had more than 70,000 nurses around the world, including in Europe, Brazil, the Middle East, and Japan.

⁜

BALANCING WORK AND FAMILY
'This morning I said goodbye to my wife and daughter'

"I DON'T THINK we had anybody say no," Dr. Murphy said about staff redeployment, even if they had to rearrange their lives, make sure their families were safe before they headed to the front lines. COVID-19, after all, went right to the core of people's home lives.

Some sent young children to stay with grandparents or other family members who could take them in, including hospitalist Grace Farris, who, before redeploying to COVID care at Mount Sinai West, delivered her children to her mother's house in Connecticut. "It's been four weeks since I've seen my kids, and I'm starting to miss them," Dr. Farris wrote in a *New York Times* Op-Ed on April 15, 2020. She detailed how she had to summon "my blackest, stoniest heart" to bear being away from her kids as well as the wide-open heart she needed to deliver humane, emotionally fraught life-and-death care in the hospital.

Others, like Joanne Hojsak, a pediatric intensive care doctor at the Mount Sinai Hospital, isolated herself at home, in the extra bedroom her family was lucky enough to have. Like so many other health care workers who were parents, it was over FaceTime that she joined her family for dinner—even though she was in the next room.

Still others retreated to hotel rooms that the health system offered. At the beginning of April, Mount Sinai Queens physician Matthew Bai decided it would be safer for his family if he were to move out during the surge. "This morning I said goodbye to my wife and my daughter for who knows how long," he said in an April 3 video diary. For weeks, he ended his wrenching shifts at the hospital by joining his wife and seventeen-month-old via video call for the nightly routine, the bedtime stories, the good night kisses.

Many, many others felt they needed to be surrounded by family, so they took every precaution from hospital to home, stripping down at their front doorway or in the garage after work and heading directly to the shower and the laundry. Then, in the morning, do it all again.

Sanam Ahmed, a critical care attending on the night shift at the Mount Sinai Hospital, was responsible, with her team, for stabilizing the sicker COVID patients, putting them on a ventilator if needed or facilitating transfer to the ICU. She was also responsible, in her other life, for her four children. "When I left my house today, I had mixed feelings," she said in an April 4 video diary. "I left my kids at home so I could go fight this war along with my colleagues."

As she left her house, she got a text from a colleague. It was a number, followed by a note: "This is the number of patients whose lives we have been saving over just the past day." Since the beginning of COVID, Dr. Ahmed and her colleagues across Mount Sinai's hospitals had treated and discharged 1,748 COVID patients by April 4.

"I feel optimistic, hopeful," said Dr. Ahmed. "As critical care physicians, this is what we've trained for, and we know we're well equipped to do it."

Gopi Patel, the Mount Sinai Hospital's epidemiologist, can read in the words of her seven-year-old daughter both gratitude for health care workers and evidence of their sacrifice. *Dear Mom and your crew,* her daughter wrote in a card from her elementary school to the hospital. *I'm thankful for you because you help people and you also take care of everyone, not just the people you like. You never give up, like if you don't know what the virus or disease is.*

"It was very sweet," said Dr. Patel, "but also a testament that there was this other piece of myself who was not getting the attention she needs. I hope you can reflect the sacrifices our health care workers made."

No matter who was waiting at home, every health care worker

sought to create that margin of safety between hospital and home, those threshold rituals. After a grueling twelve-hour shift in which one patient died and two more neared death, pulmonologist Umesh Gidwani captured his thoughts in a video diary, his cap askew and his eyes weary. "Now," he said, "I'm going to go home, have a quick shower, hopefully scrub the coronavirus off my body if not off my soul, and sit down for dinner with the family."

8 | THE MEDICAL EDUCATION OF A LIFETIME

'It will make me a more compassionate doctor'

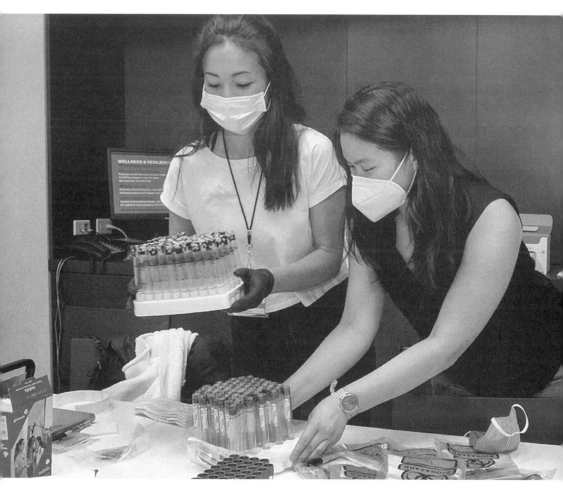

Medical and graduate research students redeployed across the health system to support clinical and scientific operations, including building the COVID-19 Biobank (above).

SOMETIMES IT TAKES a medical student—someone smart and observant, both an insider and an outsider to the long-standing health care system—to see things differently. Mount Sinai had just received a large order of much-needed face shields, some 750,000, which would go a long way toward providing PPE peace of mind. The laborious task of putting together the shields fell, as a number of tasks were starting to do, to an energized and well-organized group of volunteers: medical students recently sidelined from classrooms and clinicals. For days, student volunteers assembled the shields, until the new fleet was ready for demonstration in front of the administrative and clinical leaders who would distribute and wear the shields.

The moment didn't go well. The shields, which usually attach at the hairline and are worn over masked faces, protect primarily the eyes. These shields appeared to have a big gap right at the eyes. "This does nothing," the clinical leaders replied.

"Everyone was really fired up because they had just spent how many thousands of dollars on these face shields that have an open square right around your eyes," said Annie Arrighi-Allisan, a then-third-year student who headed the PPE task force with classmate Stephen Russell, who led the face shield effort. "It protected everything but where you wanted to protect most."

Amid the furor, she got a call from Mr. Russell, asking her to join him at the C-suite to meet with the leaders about the shields. "Stephen comes into the room, and he puts the face shield on a different way," Ms. Arrighi-Allisan narrated. "He said, 'You're not supposed to have it here. You're supposed to have it way back on the crown of your head like this.'" He demonstrated. While "it looked absurd and I could see why no one thought to put it on like that," she said, that was in fact the correct way to wear it. The face shield did, as it turned out, cover the eyes.

"Everyone is freaking out because they think that this has all been for nothing, and it just takes one really bright medical student to say, 'Actually, I think you just have it on wrong,'" Ms. Arrighi-Allisan said. One more improvement Mr. Russell added: building an additional strip of padding into the face shield assembly to protect against chafing.

"That was a real theme throughout COVID," said Ms. Arrighi-Allisan, who was on her neurology rotation when COVID hit. "Everyone wanted to help, and everyone was looking for leaders, essentially, on every level."

MARCH 15, 2020—Clerkships and clinical rotations at the Icahn School of Medicine, third- and fourth-year medical students training directly in hospitals, were cancelled for the rest of the academic year. In-person classes for first- and second-year students had already ended. All learning was transitioning online. Students' lives were suddenly upended, plans for the future on hold. They would, for the first time in forever, have time on their hands.

MARCH 16, 2020—Into this state of uncertainty and anxiety—and not used to sitting around, even for a day—a group of Mount Sinai medical students set up a meeting with their school's leadership, learned the ins and outs of the health system's extraordinary needs, and quickly created the COVID-19 Student WorkForce to bolster physicians, staff, researchers, and hospital operations in any way they could. Three days later, on March 19, tasks in hand, students began fanning out across the health system, in person or virtually, in their newly defined volunteer roles.

The WorkForce, which was established and run entirely by students, set up seven key task forces to support Mount Sinai's most pressing needs. The personal protective equipment task force, for example, helped manage PPE supply and delivery throughout the health system. Led by Ms. Arrighi-Allisan and Mr. Russell, the task force coordinated with Mount Sinai's Environmental Health Services on PPE needs and regulations, and, on the other side, connected with many individuals and groups who wanted to donate or make such equipment. That might include a dentist's office looking to donate N95 masks, or a local manufacturer looking to retool equipment to make surgical masks. The task force matched solution to need down to the last detail, including connecting Mandarin-speaking students directly to suppliers in China.

Students also served as runners, making deliveries and unpacking shipments to disseminate to hospitals, with a constant eye on how deep into the hospitals they could go and still maintain their safety. "The students loved it because they were involved and helping out," said Ms. Arrighi-Allisan. "They felt like they were actually *doing* something, delivering these potentially life-saving items. You give med students a task, and you know they're going to get it done."

Meantime, students on the pharmacy task force helped manage drug supplies and get them where they were needed, including helping to resolve medication supply shortfalls. The administrative task force handled remote medical scribe work, reprogrammed tablets in patient rooms so families could teleconference, and helped streamline inventorying of PPE. The morale task force coordinated meal deliveries to students and staff, distributed health kits to students who were sick, and fostered a sense of community—a vital part of medical school—online while students could not gather in person. On the telehealth task force, some three hundred student volunteers called patients with test results, called hospitalized COVID-19 patients to gather emergency contact information, and triaged PATCH-24, the palliative care hotline. The labs task force assisted in COVID-related research efforts, including working with the departments of microbiology and pathology to manage more than 500 requests for serum antibody testing. And the operations task force joined the enormous mobilization of resources across the health system. They assembled and delivered vital equipment, including retrofitting donated home breathing devices into patient ventilators, and helped on the operational side of clinical trials.

In the first week, with hundreds of COVID patients in Mount Sinai hospitals and a steep rise expected, student volunteers put in 947 hours. By the time the operation was up and running fully, the volunteer student workforce would commit 2,277 hours per week, on average. "One big reason we had such a great volunteer turnout is because Sinai students are so invested in patient care and wanting to be a part of the team," said Rohini Bahethi, a third-year student at the time and a task force leader. "It was frustrating to feel sidelined while so many of our resident friends who we worked closely with were out on the front lines, oftentimes redeployed into ICUs. Their stories cut deep. It was just death after death after death. A lot of students were like, 'How can we help?'"

Mount Sinai heeded the Association of American Medical Colleges' recommendation that students not engage in direct contact with patients, though the association did encourage students to adopt "innovative approaches" to their role in the solution.

"Working together in the way we did, we were able to do more collectively than any of us had done previously," said James Blum, who helped lead the workforce remotely from his temporary home in Cambridge, Massachusetts, where he was augmenting his medical degree with a degree in public policy from Harvard's Kennedy School. "The good thing and the bad thing about a crisis is that it collapses all sorts of normal structure. The positive here was that we were able to have impact that might not normally have been expected from the students."

In the first three months, student volunteers had contributed 29,602 hours to Mount Sinai's COVID relief effort. They shared their blueprint in a detailed paper, subtitled "A Model for Rapid Response in Emergency Preparedness," in *Academic Medicine*, for other students and schools facing their own pandemic—or any future—crisis.

"The fact that you have students sitting at the table, a virtual table, involved in conversations about how the health system is responding is absolutely unprecedented," said third-year student Charles Sanky, who volunteered on the telemedicine team and was tapped for a leadership role in coordinating the convalescent plasma program and tocilizumab clinical trials. "But what it shows is that you have individuals in our institution's leadership who recognize what people bring and empower them to contribute. That allows us to think outside the box, to respond in a way that isn't bound by how we've been doing things all along."

APRIL 4, 2020—As New York's COVID population was rising to an as-yet-unknown peak and there was a clamor for more health care workers, Governor Cuomo issued an executive order allowing medical students who were eligible for graduation in a matter of weeks to immediately begin practicing in New York. On April 15, 19 fourth-year Mount Sinai medical students graduated one month early and began their careers as doctors. They were joined by 10 students graduating from other medical schools who had "matched" at Mount Sinai, meaning they had secured residencies there upon graduation.

At first, the idea was that Medical Corps doctors would do everything except go into COVID patients' rooms. "I thought they would be an extra pair of eyes and ears, an extra pair of hands for the resident teams, to improve the resident team experience while giving the graduates hands-on intern-level experience," said Adriane Malone, a hematologist-oncologist who oversaw the program as senior associate dean for graduate medical education. "They wrote progress notes, ordered medications, helped with discharging and calling consults. They helped facilitate communication with patients and families. They did mostly behind-the-scenes type of work and really helped decompress their assigned teams."

As the young doctors' experience level rose, so, too, did their eagerness to get closer to the front lines. While the need for direct COVID care was, mercifully, dropping, Dr. Malone and the administrative team moved the new doctors to positions in the ED, doing triage or preoperative work, and to general medicine teams working with non-COVID patients. Eventually, some were called in where needed on COVID wards. "It really gave them a boot camp prior to internship," said Dr. Malone.

Olamide Omidele planned to step into his role as a urology resident after graduation but instead got to work a month early on the floors of the Mount Sinai Hospital. He began behind the scenes, supporting the teams, but his work evolved to frontline COVID care. "I feel we grew up quickly," he said. "These were some of the sickest patients I have ever seen."

Reflecting almost a year later on his experience, Dr. Omidele's takeaway is twofold. "First, I hope this never happens again," he said. "It was a great, great tragedy. But from a physician's perspective, I feel like if this does happen again, we'll be more prepared. It showed the resilience of the health care community, that we're willing to take on any challenge at any time."

Taking on the greatest challenge in a century, after all, was what Medical Corps doctors had signed on for. "These extremely committed medical students chose to drop themselves in at the peak of a pandemic without really knowing what to expect," said David Thomas, vice chair of education for the department of medicine. 'They had to learn how to work in a hospital while adjusting to a constantly evolving situation. They made me proud every day."

⁜

SUPPORTING STUDENTS THROUGH UNPRECEDENTED CHALLENGES
'Everything was in jeopardy'

THE ROAD TO BECOMING a doctor is a long one, with prescribed milestones along the way. Four years of medical school followed by three or four years of residency, even more for surgeons. Many Mount Sinai students combine their med school training with other professional education, including in public health or biomedical research. So the disruption of key guideposts in that training, with clinical rotations paused and classroom learning moving online, threatened the path that students had been envisioning, often for most of their lives.

"Everything was in jeopardy," said David Muller, dean for undergraduate medical education. "Their future, their goals, what they wanted to accomplish."

For many students, that abstract threat was compounded by very real challenges of the pandemic, the grief, anxiety, and economic insecurity that came as family members fell ill with or died of COVID, faced risks as essential workers, or lost jobs, livelihoods. The pandemic, as it did in so many other ways, seemed to exacerbate inequities here, too, with students whose families were more vulnerable appearing to suffer disproportionately.

"It was terrifying and heartbreaking," said Dr. Muller. "We're reasonably well-equipped to get a student through medical school, even if they're struggling. But in the setting of all this, there were just enormous gaps. What helped us was our students' willingness to share their concerns with us and be vulnerable." That enabled the school to put responsive academic and mental health supports in place, even on an "ad hoc" basis, Dr. Muller acknowledged.

Students struggled with all manner of unpredictability and loss. Julie Byrnes, who was in her first year of the MD/MPH program when COVID hit, lost her adoptive mother to COVID-19. She struggled with balancing school and, first, her mother's care, then the grief over losing her. "I'm definitely struggling—I am still in mourning," Ms. Byrnes told Mount Sinai's "COVID Memories" project. "I'm trying to stay grounded. I'm grateful to be in school now, learning useful information to hopefully help prevent this from ever getting so bad again."

One thing she learned, both in class and from searing personal experience, was how anathema it was for people to die alone, separated from family. She had just taken a medical anthropology class as part of the public health program and drew deep lessons about the evolutionary human need to care and grieve together rather than apart. She was able, as a medical student, to visit her mother in her final moments in palliative care, but Ms. Byrnes did not get to spend all the time together that she wished they could have. And she knew that she was fortunate, that most families did not get the chance to say goodbye. "That haunts me," she said.

STUDENTS SHELTERED in place in student housing and apartments, anxious about their health, their studies, their parents. Some enthusiastically volunteered to assemble and deliver PPE, put together ventilators, deliver patient test results. Others were sick themselves with COVID or caring for family members who were. But they were all still *students*, still in the Icahn School of Medicine's charge, still pursuing their medical education.

"We forced ourselves very early on to articulate guiding principles," said Dr. Muller. "When you're putting out—I don't know—twenty fires a day, if you don't have an overarching goal in mind, or a guiding principle to take you through the process, it's very easy to veer off track." While there might have been a little veering in the earliest turbulent days, Dr. Muller would go on to reflect six months after the surge that the school hewed successfully to its guiding principles and that they were, in the main, the right ones. They included:

- *Ensuring the safety of students, faculty, staff, and patients.* This meant the school transitioned to remote work and learning, paused clinical rotations, brought students home from study overseas, and created a highly active infection prevention team. "This was a public health crisis, and suddenly student health, physical health—we always talk about wellness, but physical health—was the central thing," said Valerie Parkas, a senior associate dean of recruitment and admission, who, with her colleague Beverly Forsyth, led infection prevention for the medical school. "We're infectious disease doctors. We knew immediately that keeping students safe needed to be one of our guiding principles. So we tightened the safety valve. Then, when we felt things were maybe a little more safe, we'd loosen the valve."

- *Recognizing that this is an evolving public health crisis and an unprecedented time in medical education.* School leaders met frequently with regional and national peers, encouraged development of the student volunteer task force, and committed to frequent and detailed communication and education on the pandemic.

- *Acknowledging the stressors students faced regarding their future and their goals, and viewing their pandemic experience through a lens of equity, access, and fairness.* Whatever support the medical school normally offered students—and Mount Sinai is known to be a supportive, progressive, and equitable place—it was amplified to meet a whole new level of need. The school provided meals while students were sheltering in place, augmented mental health support with telehealth visits, and worked closely with students to keep them on track to graduation, normally a very regimented process and now facing upheaval.

- *Meeting medical education program objectives and governing requirements.* Despite the exigency, this was still a medical school, responsible for the education of future doctors. Administrators had to ensure that the changes in processes and programming were done in concert with governing bodies and accrediting organizations.

Drs. Muller and Parkas, and other Mount Sinai leaders, together with colleagues at Columbia University Vagelos College of Physicians and Surgeons, Weill Cornell Medical College, and Albert Einstein College of Medicine, wrote up these principles and published them so others could learn from how New York City medical schools navigated the extraordinary crisis that hit them first and hit them hardest.

IF THERE WAS one consistency across the span of students' experiences, it was that the pandemic would indelibly shape the doctors they will go on to become.

For Charles Sanky, who still vividly recalls hearing ambulances streaming by day and night from his student apartment across from the hospital and feeling powerless to help, the pandemic reignited his commitment to a career in emergency medicine. "I knew that I wanted to go into emergency medicine, but this really reminded me of why," said recently graduated Dr. Sanky, speaking in 2021 as an emergency medicine resident at Mount Sinai. "Emergency medicine physicians always work with an all-hands-on-deck approach. You need to prioritize what you see, triage, and do everything in your power to help as many people as possible. That is a mindset everyone was using during this time."

More than that, he said, emergency medicine, at the front lines of health care provision, offers a window into the strengths and weaknesses of our health systems. Even as Mount Sinai rose to the crisis at hand, one of the pandemic takeaways, as Dr. Sanky saw it, was that the health care system as a whole was not designed to be *prepared.* "We operate at just-in-time capacity, and any time that we have extra it's seen as waste," he said. "We need to think much more about how we design systems that are able, nimble, resilient, and ready to handle everything that comes our way. This requires us to seriously think about the political, financial, regulatory, and cultural forces that stop us from actually responding to any threat."

Annie Arrighi-Allisan learned the importance of saying no, of invoking the safety and well-being of student volunteers in the face of such dire need. *Could the students put in more hours, get closer to clinical floors?* "One of the most difficult parts of the job was realizing that there were people in trouble who needed things, but the people delivering those things needed their own help—they weren't necessarily able to just do 36-hour shifts in a row," she said. "What that taught me about leadership is that it's not just about directing people. It's also about helping them to draw boundaries.

"You want to save people, make patients safer, do quality research, stop the pandemic. But in the meantime, you have to take care of the individual people" in your charge, she said, meaning health care workers, or, in her case, medical student volunteers.

Olamide Omidele, who believes that medicine is the ultimate team sport, said of the earliest days of his career, spent caring for COVID patients and caring for the people caring for COVID patients, "It will make me a more compassionate doctor. I saw patients, the whole hospital system pushed to the brink, and I saw physicians and nurses give everything to fight back this crisis. There was a lot of grit and determination."

For James Blum, while he became a more knowledgeable doctor during the pandemic—learning about infectious disease and about how health systems operate in crisis—he also became a more humble doctor. "This made me more humble about what we don't know and all that science continues to teach us, how knowledge has continued to evolve," said Dr. Blum, who in 2021 began a residency in emergency medicine at Boston Medical Center. "I feel more comfortable accepting what I don't know or what is out of my control and leading from a position of uncertainty, a position of continuing to learn more."

IN THE MIDST of the pandemic, in the 2021 application cycle, Mount Sinai saw a 26 percent rise in med school applications from the year before. Nationwide, the average increase in med school applications was 18 percent, compared with a usual year-over-year rise of about 3 percent. David Muller cautioned against reading too much into these numbers. Applications for selective colleges rose, too, with a number of factors at play (including changing admissions criteria). Online processes may have lowered barriers and freed up time for students to complete more applications. Or perhaps acquiring skills and knowledge in an uncertain world looked like the best move for people in transition.

Still, some see the rise in medical school applications as an inspiration to action, a call to duty. Says Geoffrey Young, Association of American Medical Colleges (AAMC) senior director for student affairs and programs, "I make an analogy to the time after 9/11, when we saw an increase in those motivated to serve this country militarily."

MARSHALING ESSENTIAL RESOURCES

'People are working 24/7, pursuing every lead'

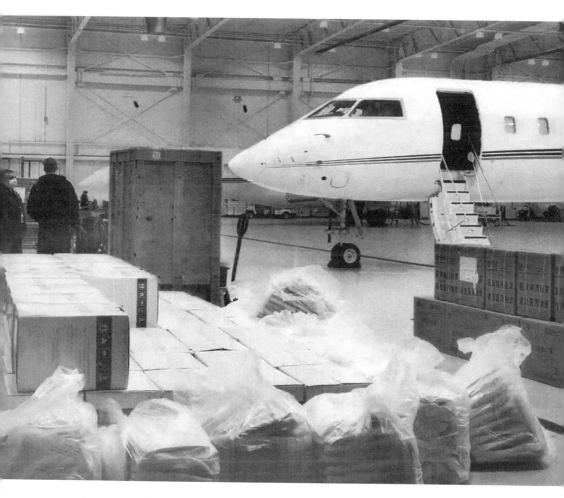

Securing supplies required a massive team effort, including a "monumental" airlift of 130,000 N95 masks from China to Mount Sinai.

WHEN BERNARD CAMINS, Mount Sinai's medical director of infection prevention, got a health alert from the Centers for Disease Control and Prevention on January 10, he immediately knew what that meant for Mount Sinai's health care workers. "I told our supply chain we need as many N95 masks as possible," he said. "I said whatever we usually order, double it."

When the mask shipment arrived in February, it was 50 percent larger, rather than double. But Dr. Camins wasn't too worried. "At that point, we had about 120,000 N95 respirators," he recalled. "And I said, 'Oh, that is a lot. We're going to be good for a while.' I was thinking we would get some patients, not knowing that, even as this was happening at the end of February, early March, the virus was already spreading in New York and no one knew it yet."

As it turned out, within five days, 30,000 of those 120,000 masks were already gone. And, with usage about to jump to 16,300 a day, the remaining 90,000 masks would not last long.

When COVID-19 hit New York with a vengeance, Mount Sinai had two critical mandates: keep staff safe and help patients breathe. This meant an exponential increase in two key resources—personal protective equipment and ventilators, whose demand rose four- or fivefold during the surge. And the need for this life-saving "stuff" was skyrocketing, not only at Mount Sinai but soon across the country and the world, just as the global supply chain was grinding to a halt, with massive shutdowns of whole economies, beginning in China.

✢

PERSONAL PROTECTIVE EQUIPMENT
'We have enough to keep you safe today'

First you put on an N95, headgear, and eye protection, goggles or an actual helmet. Then you wash your hands, put on a first pair of gloves, then a gown, then another pair of gloves. It takes three to four minutes to put on the gear. We're doing this between rooms. We're constantly washing our hands, which are so raw, dry, and cracked. We're wearing an N95 mask for twelve, fourteen hours in a day. It's rubbing constantly

on your skin. The bridge of your nose and portions of your face would be completely raw. You develop acne from the masks—they call it maskne. You're sweating because you're constantly in all this gear, and it's heavy. As austere as the gear was, you feel like you were protected.

—GLEN CHUN, *pulmonologist, the Mount Sinai Hospital*

————

YOU CANNOT TELL the story of the COVID-19 pandemic without telling the story of personal protective equipment. Gowns, gloves, goggles, surgical masks, and, most dearly, the health care-grade N95 respirators. "It became part of our everyday vernacular, this concept of donning and doffing of PPE," said Dr. Chun. "It's now an acronym that's part of the everyday language."

It was hot, took a long time to put on, and could alienate health care workers from patients and one another. It left noses and hands raw and bloody, and deepened the exhaustion of weary health care workers. But PPE saved lives. China had learned that the hard way. "The early experience in China was harrowing, and a number of providers were afflicted by and died from COVID," said Charles Powell, Mount Sinai's head pulmonologist who was in contact early on with his colleagues in China. Health care workers there were initially caught off guard by the virulent spread of the virus and hampered by manufacturing shutdowns. "However, soon after, there was a strict implementation of protocols to use PPE and isolate patients accordingly, and the number of infected health care personnel went way, way, way down. That was Lesson One: that health care providers can be safe if they use appropriate PPE."

Before COVID-19, N95 masks were hardly the stuff of legend. The ones Mount Sinai used were primarily 3M 1860s, utilitarian-looking circular masks in hospital-teal. They were pressed into service on the relatively infrequent occasion that a patient came to the hospital with or suspected of having an infectious disease, such as tuberculosis, something easily transmitted through the air. Pre-COVID, clinicians across the Mount Sinai Health System used, on average, 653 N95 masks each day. Each of those uses could be fleeting, because the masks were disposable, thrown away after each episode of use. Clinicians could go through a whole box on a single patient.

During COVID, so much changed for the humble N95, except for the fact that the mask still blocked 95 percent of airborne particulate. With supply chain interruptions, the shape of the mask would change as different vendors came on board—round, duckbill, oval. At first it was to be used only in aerosol-generating procedures, such as intubation or cardiopulmonary resuscitation, and not in regular care of COVID patients. But soon, it became clear that the condition of COVID patients could plummet so quickly that intubation or CPR might be needed at any moment, so all staff treating COVID patients should wear N95s. Later, it was determined that clinicians performing aerosol-generating procedures even on non-COVID patients should wear N95s out of an abundance of caution.

And the mask's one-and-done status was changed to reflect the frequency of use and scarcity of the resource. Mount Sinai clinicians were asked to wear the same N95 for repeated encounters with patients, either taking it off and storing it safely in between encounters or leaving it on for the duration—often, for the whole day. Mount Sinai health care workers would run through 16,360 N95 masks a day at the virus's peak.

The increased use of other pieces of PPE was just as staggering. Surgical mask use rose from 11,198 a day pre-COVID to 54,900 during the surge. Eye protection went from 366 pieces daily pre-pandemic, up to more than 6,000 daily in March and April. Mount Sinai normally went through 80,000 gowns a month. At the height of the pandemic, hospitals were using nearly 30,000 gowns *a day*.

Soaring need came just as the global supply chain was interrupted. In an ongoing effort to drive down costs in the low-margin business of health care, half of the world's PPE manufacturing had shifted to China. When the virus first ravaged Wuhan and the province went into strict lockdown, factories shut down across China. When they ramped back up shortly thereafter, Chinese authorities held fast to those resources. At the same time, other governments began restricting their own exports of PPE, right when health care workers around the world were all clamoring for it.

So at Mount Sinai, along with other hospitals across New York City, Washington State, California, and other forward-looking regions across the country and across the world, the hunt was on. At Mount Sinai, leads poured in from all corners of the organization, from employees and their family members, from trustees, from the community. Staff from purchasing and supply chain were following leads, nudging vendors, making cold calls around the clock. If someone needed to place an order at midnight Saturday, when China was open, a buyer on standby would write a purchase order then and there. Midnight Saturday.

"No one was unavailable, no one was standoffish," said Mr. Maceda, who came into his job as head of supply chain on March 1. "I was talking to other VPs and other directors at eleven at night on Saturdays. It was 24/7 on every level, it truly was everybody."

One Mount Sinai staffer drove to a specialized lab in Ohio to expedite testing of a recent new mask candidate. The health system began sourcing face shields from Bushwick, Brooklyn, and helped dozens of small businesses across the tri-state area become viable suppliers. Dr. Camins worked with a Boston-based greeting-card company branching out into hospital gowns to fix an initial prototype that left the back exposed and was not flexible enough for clinical movement. "Rather than just moving on, they actually asked us, 'Well, how do we make this better?' So I gave them advice," said Dr. Camins, noting that the resulting gowns were approved and purchased by Mount Sinai.

MEANWHILE, on the floors, PPE was a constant source of anxiety. That tension amplified following the death of Kious Kelly, the nurse at Mount Sinai West who was believed to be the first health care worker to die in New York. His nursing colleagues expressed fear and frustration over the availability of protective gear.

Getting and keeping PPE, tracking it, distributing it—that was one challenge. Another was communicating to staff different messages at once about PPE, one of the greatest sources of anxiety of the whole pandemic. As feverishly as it came in, PPE went out, so pressing and constant was the need. At the end of March, Mount Sinai had about a week's worth of PPE on hand—a threshold that it never dipped below. That was a scary prospect, one week's worth, but, at the same time, people were moving heaven and earth to source and secure it. And Mount Sinai leadership laid down a commitment never to run out.

"We could not, under any circumstances, have a situation where somebody didn't have what they needed," said Jeremy Boal, who headed the health system's employee communications during the pandemic. "But we never said, 'Everything's going to be fine. You don't have to worry.' Ever."

In email blasts, he and Dr. LoPachin, whose name and voice were on the daily emails, tried to communicate two equally true things. "One is, we don't have massive quantities," Dr. Boal explained. "We have enough to keep you safe today and for the next week. We're going to be transparent with you about that." And the second true thing: "At the same time, we're going to give insight into just how hard the entire organization is working to protect you, pursuing every lead. You need to know that Board members are putting their own money on the line. That jets are being commandeered to fly to China to pull equipment off of a landing strip. That people are working 24/7, pursuing every lead to get you what you need."

MARCH 27, 3 A.M., TETERBORO AIRPORT—Two airplanes touched down twelve miles from midtown Manhattan carrying 130,000 N95 masks from Nanjing, China, nearly doubling Mount Sinai's supply, with another 350,000 on their way.

The story of the overnight transcontinental PPE mission began nearly two years earlier, when Mount Sinai entered into a consultative partnership with Taikang Nanjing International Medical Center, a few hundred miles from Wuhan. It is one of several global partnerships Mount Sinai has with medical centers around the world who want to tap Sinai's expertise in clinical care. When the virus hit Wuhan in January, Mount Sinai reached out to the Nanjing hospital and sent supplies.

When the virus had crested in China and production there ramped back up in March, the Nanjing hospital secured 500,000 N95s and 1.2 million surgical masks to send to Mount Sinai. But flight restrictions in China and internationally made it impossible to get the masks to New York.

Impossible, that is, until Richard Friedman, co-chair of the Mount Sinai Boards of Trustees, got involved. When he learned from Mount Sinai CEO Ken Davis that the PPE bound for Mount Sinai was stuck on a tarmac, Mr. Friedman remembered back to 9/11, when grounded air travel prevented him from getting home to New York from Japan. The Goldman Sachs executive did then what he was about to do now— make a phone call to see if Warren Buffet's company, NetJets, could scramble some planes and airlift the PPE. "Literally, within three to five minutes, NetJets was cleared to send two [Bombardier] Global 6000s," said Mr. Friedman.

After a flurry of phone calls to gain necessary approvals, the NetJets planes flew from Alaska to China. When they arrived, four pilots from each plane found pallets of masks originally packed for a cargo jet and unbundled the cargo, box by box, to load into the newly arrived passenger planes. Only 130,000 of the 500,000 could fit, but that would be enough to double Mount Sinai's supply.

Mr. Friedman worked through the night with leaders at Nanjing's airport to get the masks through customs, and at 3 a.m., the masks landed at Teterboro Airport. "Everything we do here is going to save a life," said Mr. Friedman, whose son was a fourth-year resident at Mount Sinai working with COVID patients. "And I could very easily personalize it. I was trying to help every single person, but there was added urgency: I've got to help my son."

The touchdown of the plane reverberated throughout Mount Sinai's health system. "That was like the Super Bowl team coming back home to their home city," said Rob Sharma, at Mount Sinai South Nassau. "Everybody was cheering that event. It was a huge relief of anxiety and tension."

While the assembled team was prepared to repeat the mission for the remaining N95s, as well as 1.2 million surgical masks, airline restrictions began to lift, and the cargo flight was okayed for transport.

In an email to staff, Dr. LoPachin wrote, "This is monumental."

WHILE THE STATE of global supply chains created huge obstacles for much of the "stuff" needed to weather the pandemic, local communities made sure that the comforting stuff of daily life—nourishment for the body and the soul, a word of thanks, a clever cloth mask—made its way to health care workers.

Donated food poured in by the ton from favorite New York restaurants, pizza parlors, bakeries. Stop & Shop delivered food by the truckload three times a week at many Mount Sinai hospitals. During the surge, about 10,000 salads were delivered each week across the seven New York City hospitals. A Long Island nursery placed carnations on every car in the Mount Sinai South Nassau parking lot one day in April. Mount Sinai Morningside hosted free haircuts for health care workers ("those of us who still have hair," noted MSM President Art Gianelli, who does not). And a local Girl Scout troop donated a carton of cookies. Community groups and individuals collected, created, and donated a seemingly endless supply of non-medical grade masks. Messages of gratitude were chalked brightly on cement sidewalks outside every Mount Sinai hospital, and nightly seven o'clock pot-banging and cheering on the streets of New York provided a moment of uplift for many weary health care workers.

✣

MACGYVERING VENTILATORS
'We designed a better mousetrap'

You can't survive without it. In healthy individuals, it's a reflex. Our brain signals the diaphragm to drop. That goes down, and the air flows into your lungs. When you exhale, your diaphragm comes up, and the air goes out. When you're perfectly healthy, your breathing doesn't mean much to you because it's something you don't think of. But for a person who develops a cardiac or lung problem, breathing becomes the most difficult thing they do in their life. Oxygen goes to every single tissue and cell of your body. If there is a lack of oxygen in your system—and that's what

> **COVID was doing to people—your organs can start to fail. It all starts from the oxygen.**
>
> —VADIM LEYKO, *respiratory therapist, Mount Sinai Brooklyn*

————

COVID CREATED RECORD demand for ventilators and other oxygen-assistive devices. Mount Sinai could have run out of ventilators, said David Reich. As the predictive models of future COVID-19 hospitalizations in New York City started to emerge in mid-March, a shortage of ventilators became a paramount concern statewide. At that time, about one in five patients admitted to a hospital with COVID-19 needed to be placed on a ventilator—a surge in demand that would surely outstrip current supply.

At the start of the pandemic, hospitals in Europe were running out of ventilators, and health systems across New York, the United States, and the world were clamoring for them. Mount Sinai furiously sourced ventilators from myriad vendors. "It was extremely gratifying as an anesthesiologist to go on a ventilator-buying spree," noted Dr. Reich.

What happens when hundreds of ventilators needing assembly come in all at once to a health system using just about every last square inch of its space for patient care? An entire floor of the Icahn School of Medicine's Levy Library, which had already been repurposed to store hospital beds, was converted into a ventilator and respiratory device assembly factory. "With assistance from volunteers and medical students, daily shipments of respiratory devices were rapidly assembled, tested and shipped out on courier trucks across the health system," Dr. Reich recalled. "We used this same approach to distribute ventilators received from the national reserve. We approximately quadrupled the number of critical care ventilators in six weeks."

Still, with no endpoint in sight, there was no assurance in March and early April that the health system wouldn't run out of ventilators. So clinicians "MacGyver'd" a solution, moving beyond traditional critical care ventilators.

On behalf of Tesla, Elon Musk had donated two hundred home ventilators, palm-sized BiPAP machines typically used for sleep apnea.

"We immediately said thank you," said Charles Powell, Mount Sinai's head pulmonologist, and then got to work "at really effective warp speed" to adapt the home ventilators to potentially support ICU patients. First, doctors had to reduce the amount of a patient's exhalation that would be released into the air, which they did by adding a filter to the exhalation port and by replacing the mask interface with an endotracheal tube to create a closed system. They then had to make sure the device could be monitored from outside the room, a necessary precaution to minimize traffic into a COVID room. These machines couldn't pump air into the lungs at very high pressure, as ventilators did, noted Hooman Poor—a level of pressure that would have been necessary for patients with stiff lungs. But, as Dr. Poor and others had already found, the respiratory distress that COVID caused didn't seem to stiffen the lungs as much as in typical ARDS.

"We took a home device, used for someone with sleep apnea, and actually MacGyver'd it, for lack of a better term, into working as a hospital critical care ventilator," said Robbie Freeman, who, as vice president of clinical innovation, was central to the team. "And we came up with ways to monitor them remotely. You can check the settings from outside the room and can make adjustments. We used these as a proof of concept with our ICU patients and it held up very well."

The around-the-clock schedule so common in the COVID era got a boost from the eighteen-hour time difference between New York and New Zealand. World-renowned sleep expert David Rapoport, a Mount Sinai pulmonologist on sabbatical in New Zealand, developed the protocol during his day, then handed it off to the New York-based team to test all day in their lab. "We were doing that type of continuous iterative cycle to build these MacGyver ventilators," said Mr. Freeman.

The team quickly shared the protocol worldwide. As it turned out, Mount Sinai did not need the ventilators in the first wave (or subsequent waves). It retained a strategic reserve for future waves and donated remaining devices to Honduras, Africa, and the Middle East, as well as to India during its pandemic crisis in spring 2021. "If we run out of ventilators, this is another type of ventilator that we could tap into," said Mr. Freeman.

In the heat of the moment—and asked to do so by New York State officials—Mount Sinai expanded options even further, investigating the potentially harrowing territory of splitting one ventilator to serve two patients. This was no easy task, with the delicacy of the settings, the fragility of the lungs, and the highly variable needs from patient to patient. "We designed a better mousetrap by working with the ICU and anesthesiology teams to address the very frightening scenario of needing to use one ventilator on more than one patient simultaneously," said Dr. Reich. "While many jury-rigged ventilator-splitting designs have been published or posted online by anesthesiology colleagues, they are inherently unsafe in that the unequal stiffness of the lungs of the patients will direct the least amount of air into the patient with the stiffest lungs."

Anesthesiologist Matthew Levin and his team solved that issue by designing and 3D-printing a needle valve that successfully captured the hairsbreadth precision needed and created a better balance between the two patients in the simulation laboratory as part of a proof-of-concept study published in the October 2020 issue of *Anesthesiology*.

Dr. Reich praised the innovation for—as was becoming more frequent for Mount Sinai during the pandemic—creating a whole new sense of what was possible. "Although," he noted, "as an anesthesiologist, I never want to use it."

DON BOYCE—who, by personality and profession, was *prepared*—made sure that Mount Sinai had strategic guidelines in place should they ever face the Solomonic decisions that colleagues in Italy's overwhelmed Lombardy region had been forced to make. With the end point unknown during New York's frightening spring spike, Mr. Boyce wanted to make sure his organization was always looking ahead. He connected the Mount Sinai emergency work group focusing on crisis standards of care with former colleagues of his from the Department of Health and Human Services, who were the country's foremost experts on the topic. And he charged the group: "I want you to think of a time down the road, be it a couple of days, a couple of weeks, a couple of months, when we're going to have more patients than we can handle, not enough beds to put them in, not enough medication to provide to them, then I want you to close your eyes and make that a hundred times worse. And then I want you to plan for that."

How do we decide who gets the next ventilator, the next dose of medication, the next oxygen tank? he asked. *How do we define a hierarchy of needs to determine as a system what we're going to do when we reach that point?* In outlining answers to those cardinal questions, Mount Sinai could deliver its workers something of a godsend if the system were forced to make such decisions. "Medical care providers would be doing so based on policy and wouldn't be forced to make personal decisions that would haunt them for the rest of their professional careers," said Mr. Boyce.

As head of critical care, Roopa Kohli Seth would have been instrumental in carrying out the protocol if things got out of hand. Many months after the first wave, the thought of enacting crisis standards of care still weighed heavily. "I can discuss it," Dr. Kohli-Seth said in a fall interview, making it clear that she would much rather not.

The better story, after all, was the *actual* story, the story to date, the one in which Mount Sinai did not have to decide during that initial unprecedented surge who should get ventilators and who would have to go without. Mount Sinai's commitment could remain in place: relentless care for all.

PART 3

THE URGENCY OF SCIENCE

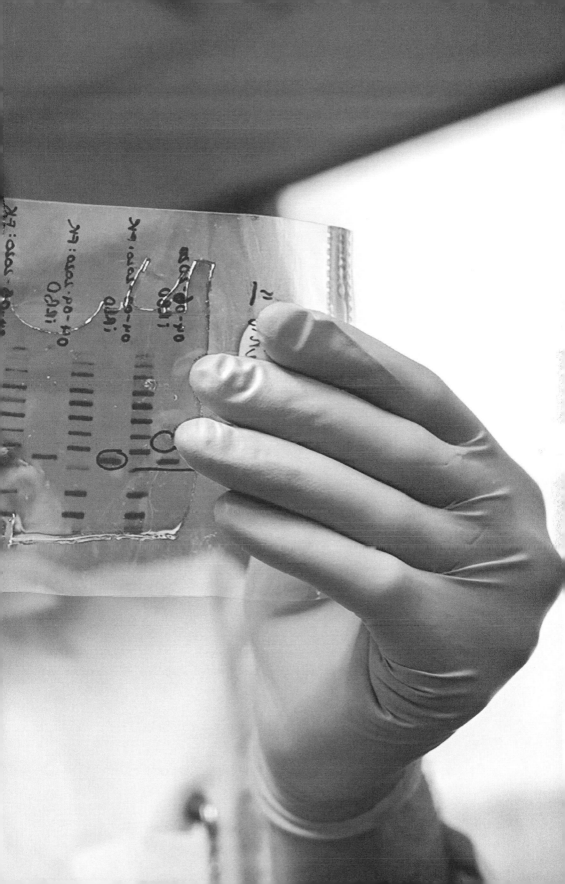

10 | SCIENCE IN THE SERVICE OF HUMANITY

'Our weapon was our science'

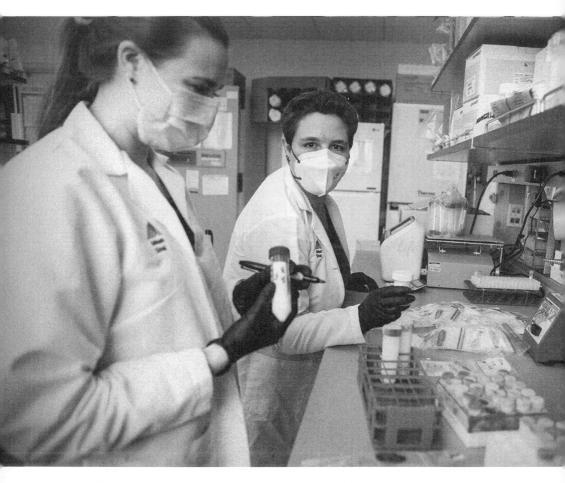

Scientists interrogating the antibody response to the novel virus included infectious disease researchers Rebecca Powell and Alisa Fox (above), and virologist Florian Krammer (previous page).

AS WITH THEIR COLLEAGUES on the front lines and behind the scenes of clinical care, Mount Sinai researchers attending to SARS-CoV-2 worked around the clock, in their case to answer essential questions about the virus, shed light on better diagnostics and potential therapies, and translate findings to patients in hours and days rather than science's usual pace of months and years. In a race against a rapidly proliferating virus, there was, simply, no time to lose.

"We had to mobilize very quickly to treat patients," said Dennis Charney, dean of the medical school. "At the same time, given that we didn't know, no one knew, how to treat this disease, we had to mobilize our scientists—our basic scientists, our translational scientists, our physician-scientists—to rapidly try to understand the disease and develop new treatments and new ways of diagnosing."

The first thing the international scientific community learned about the virus was that it was closely related to SARS-CoV-1, the source of another 21st-century epidemic and a virus that stoked fear in the hearts of many a Mount Sinai virologist. This iteration of SARS rapidly outpaced the first, besieging its virus-naive human hosts with a barrage of symptoms—some expected, some surprising. It was stubbornly complicated to track and to treat, and there was an urgent need to better understand where it was lurking and how it was spreading. Mount Sinai's long-standing expertise in and collaborative platforms for pathogen surveillance and pandemic preparedness were pressed into service immediately to help deliver answers.

The pandemic demanded exploration both on the molecular level, understanding a tiny virus that was wreaking havoc on the human body, and on the population level, where big data could reveal patterns and suggest solutions. Mount Sinai mobilized an army of redeployed researchers into a COVID-19 blood banking project whose yield from a burgeoning patient population greatly amplified previous sample collection, and which provided a vital repository for scientists to study, both amid the urgency of the pandemic and into the future.

"We felt we were in a time of war, and our weapon was our science," said Miriam Merad, who is one of the world's leading experts in the human immune system and who was involved in SARS-CoV-2 science on a number of fronts, including mobilizing researchers for the biobank collection.

✢

A MEDICAL SCHOOL BORN OF A HOSPITAL

'Science in the service of solving problems of disease'

In this rapidly changing world, the medical sciences advance so swiftly that a teaching and research hospital which lags behind is soon obsolete. Extensive research programs must be continued to develop new drugs, new techniques, new equipment. A broad, ever-expanding teaching program is required to communicate new knowledge and new techniques to the professional men and women who administer them for the benefit of patients. We at Mount Sinai are thus committed to change ... to meet the growing needs of our community, to move ever forward.

—*Mount Sinai program, dedication of Esther and Joseph Klingenstein Clinical Center, November 1962*

———

FROM THE START, the school of medicine at Mount Sinai and its research mandate were different from most medical schools. Rather than arising out of a university, as most schools were, Mount Sinai's school of medicine was created by the hospital itself. In the 1950s, the century-old Mount Sinai Hospital on the Upper East Side of Manhattan was well regarded for its clinical care and received the most federal funding for clinical research of any stand-alone hospital.

But medical leaders knew that the institution had to take a profound step forward if it wanted to stay at the top of its game. To keep pace at the forefront of clinical care, the hospital had to be affiliated with a medical school, a place to conduct rigorous science on new horizons and to train generations of students to continually carry biomedical science into the future. After an exhaustive search of New York universities to partner with, and amid a few tentative partnerships that failed to pan out, the Mount Sinai Hospital decided to open its own medical school, the Mount Sinai School of Medicine, chartered by the New York State Board of Regents in 1963. The medical school and the hospital are guided by a single board of trustees, which Mount Sinai's leadership believes is integral to the seamless partnership between the school and the hospitals.

The medical school envisioned by one of its principal founders, pathologist Hans Popper, would excel in research at both ends of the spectrum. "As we raise the magnification, the similarity of the biologic processes in all living organisms becomes apparent," he wrote in 1965, in the school's infancy. "Extrapolations can be made, for example, from bacterial and viral genetics to diseases in humans."

At the same time, Dr. Popper planned a medical school that would "relate to the city of New York as a whole, not only to the great cultural center but also to the large masses of people of all walks of life, all colors, races or creeds. The center must be dedicated not only to some level of care of the masses in the large metropolis but rather to search for methods to cover adequately large groups of populations in the future setting of medicine."

The Mount Sinai School of Medicine became New York City's seventh medical school when it opened in 1968 to 59 students in a remodeled bus garage, next to the Mount Sinai Hospital.

One of the first students to attend, in the school's second-ever class, was a young Yale graduate, Kenneth Davis, now the Mount Sinai Health System's CEO, who was drawn to the new school's mission. Speaking on the occasion of the school's fiftieth anniversary, Dr. Davis, who from 2003 to 2007 was dean of the school as well as CEO of the health system, said: "It was very clear that this was not a university with a medical school—this was a *hospital*. A hospital like this, which had a tradition of doing research, valued science. But it valued science for the sake of facilitating patient care, understanding diagnoses, understanding pathophysiology. It was a place that put science in the service of solving problems of disease. What differentiates us is when we think about what we want to study, we study the places where we can have a huge therapeutic consequence."

"Our mission is clear," said Dennis Charney, who has been dean since 2007. "Mount Sinai science leads to new therapeutics for patients who need them most." Indeed, both Drs. Davis and Charney have conducted groundbreaking research that translated into therapies for diseases that include Alzheimer's disease and treatment-resistant depression.

Fast forward to the greatest pandemic in a century, and that founding mission was sharply in evidence, with researchers interrogating the science to advance treatments in real time, in urgent time, in pandemic time. "We were about to surge," said Dr. Davis, setting the scene at the brink of the first wave. "As soon as we began to see these COVID patients, our doctors—who are physician-scientists—are already thinking, What's the best thing to do?"

✝

COVID RESEARCH: AN OVERVIEW

'It is important to get as much data as possible'

THROUGHOUT THE PANDEMIC, Mount Sinai researchers published nearly 800 articles in peer-reviewed journals, which were cited more than 16,600 times by other scientists. Thanks to Mount Sinai virologists, the medical community came to know more about antibody production, promising therapeutics, and potential vaccine options to increase global access. Mount Sinai science led to an understanding of where in the world New York's brutal first-wave came from and how it spread. Observation and action by Mount Sinai physician-scientists, in conjunction with data scientists, lent insight into how COVID-19 was causing dangerous clotting and what should be done about it. Mount Sinai immunologists contributed findings to the search for targeted therapies to quell the brutal, and often fatal, inflammatory storm that can accompany the illness.

The lion's share of Mount Sinai's scientific investigations spanned a few key areas of study, most especially microbiology, as well as pathology, immunology, and genetic and genomic science, which will be detailed in this section, and cardiovascular medicine and science, explored earlier, in Chapter 3.

But Mount Sinai's SARS-CoV-2 research was certainly wide-ranging, including: studying breast milk in women who have recovered from COVID-19 for the presence of antibodies; describing viral sanctuaries in the gastrointestinal tract of recovered COVID-19 patients, prompting a further look at repurposing medicines used to treat inflammatory bowel disease (IBD) to now treat COVID-19; and finding asymptomatic COVID-19 transmission among Marine recruits under strict quarantine, which could have implications for monitoring other large groups of young people, for instance, in schools and colleges.

In one of Mount Sinai's earliest scientific findings, Adam Bernheim and Michael Chung became the first U.S. radiologists to define key characteristics of COVID 19 on a CT scan, including the now-well-known ground-glass opacities. Working with data gathered very early in the outbreak from colleagues in China, the Mount Sinai radiologists demonstrated that thoracic imaging—radiology and CT scans—can play a complementary role to PCR testing in the diagnosis, prognosis, and triaging of patients with COVID-19, even more so when augmented by artificial intelligence. In those early days, amid runaway spread and scarce testing, the imaging discovery was thought to be another promising tool to speed evaluation and testing. In the first ten months following the publication of the studies, as the pandemic rampaged across the United States and the world, the radiologists' seminal findings were cited more than 1,000 times by fellow scientists.

To get the latest promising treatments to its patients, Mount Sinai offered as many clinical trials as it could, particularly in the areas of prevention and treatment. That included COVID-19 clinical trials for hyperimmune globulin (essentially, purified antibodies from convalescent plasma) and monoclonal antibodies; a number of trials targeting different pathways of the immune system to block the dangerous inflammation that COVID can create; and, early in the pandemic, trials for mesenchymal stem cell transplants. Mount Sinai also enrolled the health system in industry vaccine trials: two trials for the mRNA vaccine made by Pfizer and one for the adenovirus-vector vaccine made by Janssen/Johnson & Johnson. The trials, noted clinical trials expert Judith Aberg, always aimed to reach underrepresented New Yorkers, particularly those hard hit by the pandemic, including Blacks and Hassidic Jews.

The range of trials also included one to see if fish oil could help patients suffering from anosmia, the loss of smell often accompanying the virus, and, in May 2021, the first large-scale prospective study to examine the impact of COVID-19 infection during pregnancy on maternal and child outcomes. "There is limited data about how COVID-19 affects moms and babies, and I think it is important to get as much data as possible," said Whitney Lieb, an OB/GYN and population health expert who was co-investigator of the study—and who gave birth to baby Jacob in July 2020. "That is why I decided to join the study."

BIOMEDICAL RESEARCH, advancement, and translation to patients is a highly regulated affair, necessarily so. In the United States, new drugs need approval from the Food and Drug Administration before they can be sold. FDA approval means a drug has been deemed safe and effective, with significant health benefits that outweigh risks. The process can be lengthy and cumbersome but adds an important measure of confidence for patients and clinicians.

The pandemic accelerated the urgency, and the urgency accelerated the approval process. In the face of widespread disease and death with no proven treatment, the FDA began to issue Emergency Use Authorization (EUA) for therapies that showed promise, even though there was not the conclusive data required for full FDA approval. An EUA, explained Dr. Aberg, "just says there may be benefits. The EUA doesn't say that there *is* benefit—but there could be benefit."

Most of COVID science that was translated to patients was authorized this way, for emergency use, including both the overwhelmingly successful vaccines whose distribution began at the end of 2020 and missteps such as hydroxychloroquine, a drug that not only failed to ease COVID symptoms but was also found to cause heart complications.

Even when studies or trials fail to pan out, when something hopeful in the end proves not to be—this is the scientific method. Going down roads that lead to cul-de-sacs or back to the road you were on before—these are necessary to build the map of biomedical progress. Some early clinical trials failed to show benefit. Others, including those investigating immunomodulation and certain measures of anticoagulation, were unable to launch when Mount Sinai's COVID-19 patient population dwindled, thankfully, after the initial surge. Other hypotheses failed to pan out. Some of the most important questions have yet to be answered, even after a year and a half of concentrated global science. *What level of antibodies is necessary for protection? Why does the immune system fail to regulate itself? What causes the lingering illness known as post-acute COVID syndrome?*

"This is how science works," said Dr. Merad. "You make a hypothesis, and then you test. You analyze how the patients are doing, and you also measure responses at the biological level. And then either you find that there is no benefit, unfortunately, or maybe you have such a strong benefit for the treatment that you can sometimes even stop the trial early. But the process remains the same: You have to test."

In the pursuit of novel science, failure *is* an option. "Failure is more than okay because it means you're pushing the envelope," said Dean Charney. "Unless failure is acceptable and collaboration is supported, you're not going to be in a place that makes the kind of difference we make for patients. Ours is a culture of innovation and entrepreneurship, just like what you hear about Apple: We want our scientists to think the impossible is possible."

This kind of research is not cheap, and Mount Sinai mobilized on that front, too. The health system made available $80 million from its budget to fund SARS-CoV-2 research. Mount Sinai scientists also received $113.6 million in COVID research funding from federal, industry, foundation, and university sources, including $40.5 million directly from the NIH. In addition, in the first six months of the pandemic, the Mount Sinai Health System raised more than $70 million for its COVID relief efforts to underwrite both the clinical response and the research effort.

÷

COLLABORATION AND CHALLENGE

'The first thing is to make sure that nobody is getting infected'

CHINA, ITALY, FRANCE, England, India, Spain, Austria, Finland, Australia, Algeria, Brazil, Vietnam. It would be hard to think of a country that Mount Sinai scientists didn't in some way partner with for COVID research, to learn from, to share first-hand information with, and to collaborate with on research into antibodies, antiviral drugs, vaccines, immunomodulation, and pathology, among other areas, as you will read in the upcoming chapters.

"Everything I learned I discuss with my colleagues all over the world," said Dr. Merad, who was constantly participating in virtual meetings, conferences, and webinars with colleagues all over the world as well as teaching classes to an international array of students, including some from her native Algeria. "The scientific community was meeting across borders from day one, and we were discussing results in a very open manner—much more so than ever before."

In a presentation on his work during COVID, virologist Adolfo Garcia-Sastre showed the desktop of his computer, which featured more than 70 folder icons, each containing a separate set of collaborators he was working with to create antivirals (University of San Francisco and the Pasteur Institute in Paris), for example, and vaccines (Vietnam, Brazil, Mexico, and more). A Spaniard, he appeared every week on Spanish media to give updates on the pandemic. Many of Mount Sinai's scientists were raised and educated outside the United States and were devoted to keeping their home countries up to date on the latest science and medicine.

While the ubiquity of Zoom and the rare momentum of the entire international scientific enterprise pointed in the same direction opened great opportunities for global collaboration, still, something was lost during a year-plus of travel bans, social distancing, and shutdowns. Cardiologist Valentin Fuster headed not only Mount Sinai

Heart in Manhattan but also the National Center for Cardiovascular Investigation in Madrid. He had been traveling to Spain every week to see patients and work with colleagues. But not during the pandemic.

"It's not the same," said Dr. Fuster, shaking his head sadly as he reflected on the extended two-dimensionality of the virtual versus the visceral.

AS IT DID ON THE CLINICAL and operational sides of health care, the pandemic also yielded a split-screen feel in the research enterprise. Those whose work could pivot to COVID and inform its science—the virologists, the immunologists, the pathologists, among others—doubled down in their labs, often working around the clock with the same sense of urgency that staff on the clinical side were feeling. Also working around the clock were data scientists, whose "labs" were essentially their computers, who could continue their research projects at home and, for some, shift their lens to the large universe of data on COVID patients now streaming into Mount Sinai hospitals. And many young staffers were redeployed to one of the backbones of the research enterprise during the pandemic: building the COVID-19 Biobank.

But for the majority of Mount Sinai's scientists, New York's COVID shutdowns extended to their labs, pausing their work from mid-March to mid-May. Eric Nestler, a neuroscientist who heads Mount Sinai's research enterprise as dean for academic and scientific affairs, had never taken more than a few days away from his research, even when he was putatively on vacation. "That eight weeks that we were closed down seemed like an eternity to me," he said. "It felt like the Earth stopped rotating."

He recalled the unsettling feeling of walking through Mount Sinai's empty corridors at closing time on March 18, seeing the darkened labs, then walking home through New York City's cavernous, deserted streets. "It was like in a post-apocalypse," he said. "I never thought in my lifetime I'd ever see anything like that. That sticks with me, and it has given me a new sense of vulnerability of not only humanity but everything associated with humanity, including our research enterprise. We're so proud of NIH-funded research in the United States—which brought us these incredible vaccines in record time. But it's really vulnerable, and we need to work very hard to preserve it."

For those who stayed in the lab, it was impossible to separate work during a pandemic from life during a pandemic (as was true, too, for clinicians). In Florian Krammer's lab, one of the microbiology labs working full-throttle on COVID research, he directed researchers and assistants to avoid commuting by public transportation during the first wave, so those outside of biking or walking distance were asked to stay home. "The first thing is to make sure that nobody is getting infected, nobody is putting themselves in harm's way," said Dr. Krammer. "If you lived in Queens or New Jersey and you have to take three subways, you [could] get exposed."

Things got easier when donations came in to cover Uber rides to work for researchers who needed them. "That helped a lot," said Dr. Krammer. "We started to order pizza and soft drinks so nobody had to go out and look for food. We made it as comfortable as possible for everybody, but that only helps to a certain degree."

Dr. Merad was acutely aware of the toll the pandemic year took on young researchers, particularly women, who were at a pivotal time in their careers and whose childcare challenges were greatly amplified during COVID. "The closure of schools and day-care centers has excluded parents of small kids from the research effort, creating two classes of scientists: those who are able to afford private care and those who are not," Dr. Merad wrote in *Nature Medicine* in a piece called "Reflections from a Mother Scientist," which advocates for, among other things, affordable, accessible childcare. "Trainees have been the most-affected group among parent scientists: unable to work at the bench, they have compromised months of research, which has caused substantial delays in their research careers and has affected their job prospects."

The steep cost of higher education and of childcare in the United States—compared to such costs in Europe and elsewhere—put additional burdens on young parents in academia, she said in a follow-up interview.

The pandemic also magnified the mission and meaning of a career in research. Those who could participate rose to meet the challenge of a lifetime, believing even deep into the overnight hours that this was what they had gone into research for. Witnessing young researchers accelerate their expertise and impact has been "one of the few great things that comes out of this pandemic," said Dr. Garcia-Sastre.

"Conducting research in the middle of a pandemic is something that they will remember all their lives and that will certainly shape their research careers," he said. "They have matured as researchers. They have worked in a spirit of collaboration and seen that they could do things together very quickly. They have translated their work into action because that's what was really needed at this moment. They have worked twenty-four hours a day, seven days a week, trying to make an impact in public health. I have a great hope for this new generation of investigators that comes after us."

11

MICROBIOLOGY: THE VIRUS HUNTERS

'How much antibody do we need to be protected?'

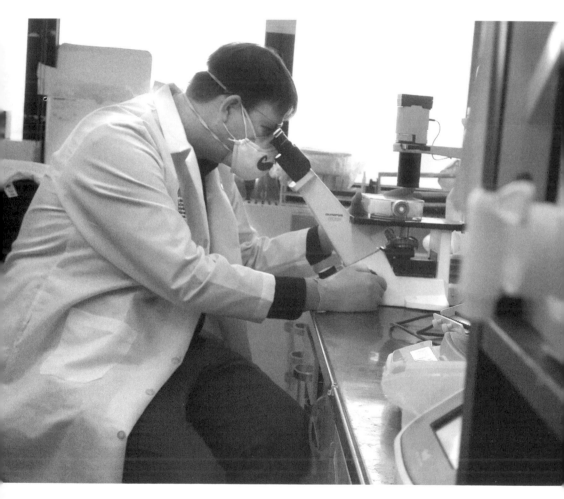

Collaborating across Mount Sinai and the world, virologist Florian Krammer developed one of the first tests to measure the level of SARS-CoV-2 antibodies in the blood.

About 25,000 cogs and machines make a single cell work, and you're made up of a trillion cells. A virus gets into one cell, and with only about seven to 12 components it completely takes over your cell, usurps all the processes, takes all the energy and resources to make more of itself. That's the nature of a virus.

—BENJAMIN TENOEVER, *professor of microbiology*

———

NEW YEAR'S EVE, DECEMBER 31, 2019—The talk of the day was of the 2020 Democratic primary polls and the upcoming presidential impeachment (not yet known as the "first impeachment"), of the season's football title games and the record-high stock markets. It was the end of a rather uneventful decade, the 2010s, albeit one quivering with high-octane populism and a sense of unease and distrust. As Michiko Kakutani wrote in *The New York Times* on December 27, "Apocalypse is not yet upon our world as the 2010s draw to an end, but there are portents of disorder."

At a New Year's Eve party on the Upper West Side, Mount Sinai virologist Florian Krammer was talking about something else: dozens of cases of pneumonias of unknown etiology that were cropping up in Wuhan, China. "I had just read about it," he recounted. "I was telling people, 'These things happen, and we're still not really prepared for a pandemic.'" On his active Twitter feed, he captioned the news out of Wuhan with a simple: "This is not good."

Ten days later, on January 10, Fudan University released the genomic sequence of the virus, confirming rumors that it was indeed a coronavirus. Dr. Krammer grew even more alarmed. "I have a lot of respect for coronaviruses," he said. This was not just any coronavirus but one that looked a lot like SARS-CoV-1. "You ask an RNA virologist when we were last close to a pandemic, they will tell you that it was in 2003 with SARS. So if you see that sequence and how closely related it is to the SARS coronavirus 1 sequence, that's when the alarm bells go off."

In the emerging virus class that he teaches, Dr. Krammer always pointed to the dangers of SARS-CoV-1, first reported in Asia, which sickened 8,096 people in 29 countries, including Canada, and killed

774, according to the CDC. The virus, as it turned out, was transmissible only by symptomatic people, so communities could respond effectively by containing those who had fever and other flu-like symptoms. A researcher in Dr. Krammer's lab, who was a boy in China during the SARS-CoV-1 outbreak, recalled having his temperature taken every morning before entering school.

SARS-CoV-2, however, had a crucial difference, one that enabled it to spread like wildfire across the world. SARS-CoV-2 was transmissible even by people who were presymptomatic or asymptomatic. It was impossible to stop the spread simply by quarantining the sick.

"This virus was the perfect one to cause more problems than normally influenza does—but not enough problems that it will be easy to identify people who are infected and then isolate them," said Dr. Garcia-Sastre, who is one of the world's leading experts on influenza and director of the Global Health and Emerging Pathogens Institute. Dr. Garcia-Sastre had been in Beijing at the beginning of the outbreak, returning home to New York the day before the virus sequence was released.

For Dr. Krammer, the fact that he kept hearing distinctions between America and Wuhan—*oh, those wet markets are so dirty, with live animals; we don't have that here*—only increased his alarm. Once SARS-CoV-2 numbers surpassed the 2003 SARS-CoV-1 numbers, which happened in the first part of February, Dr. Krammer thought, "This cannot be stopped anymore."

✢

THE MACRO IMPACT OF MICROBIOLOGY
'At Sinai there are already bridges'

Although hardly as predictable as the tides, the recurrence of pandemics is predictable, if the record of the last 400 years is any guide to the future.

—EDWIN D. KILBOURNE, *founding chair of Mount Sinai's microbiology department, writing in 1976*

It might seem unusual for people who don't work in virology or epidemiology, but we have a pandemic about every twenty-five years. They keep coming. They might actually speed up in the future because of habitat destruction, because of more farming, more animals, and climate change. That drives the chances up. It's not an unusual thing—it's a natural thing.

—FLORIAN KRAMMER, *professor of microbiology, speaking in 2020*

MOUNT SINAI'S STORIED microbiology department, which, with more than 200 scientists, is one of the most prestigious and productive in the country, specializes in RNA-containing viruses, particularly influenza viruses. Department chair Peter Palese is a pioneer in the field, and his ability to attract to Mount Sinai excellent postdoctoral fellows over the years—including Drs. Krammer and Garcia-Sastre—is legendary. Dr. Palese established the first genetic maps for influenza A, B, and C viruses, identified the function of several viral genes, and defined the mechanism of neuraminidase inhibitors, a class of drugs that are now FDA-approved antivirals. He has also deepened the world's understanding of the deadly pandemic virus that caused the worldwide 1918 Spanish flu. A team that included Drs. Palese, Garcia-Sastre, and fellow Mount Sinai micro biologist Christopher Basler reconstructed the virus strain in the laboratory using sequences obtained from material retrieved from people who died in that pandemic.

Influenza is prevalent the world over and is no stranger to jumping species, so it has great pandemic potential. Mount Sinai virologists have had their eyes on preventing pandemics—especially those coming from influenza—since the department was established in the 1960s. The founding department chair, Edwin Kilbourne, who created the first genetically engineered vaccine in 1969, for influenza, wrote in his 1976 *New York Times* Op-Ed: "World-wide epidemics, or pandemics, of influenza have marked the end of every decade since the 1940's—at intervals of exactly eleven years 1946, 1957 and 1968. A perhaps simplistic reading of this immediate past tells us that 11 plus

1968 is 1979, and urgently suggests that those concerned with the public health had best plan without further delay for an imminent natural disaster."

In the years that followed, epidemics (of both influenza and other diseases) included the global HIV/AIDS epidemic, particularly rampant in the 1980s and 1990s; the first iteration of SARS coronavirus in 2003; and the 2009 H1N1 flu pandemic. Icahn Mount Sinai has several centers and programs dedicated to surveilling viruses (again, largely influenza) around the world and studying their pathogenesis, including virus-host interactions, as well as to vaccine and antiviral drug development. During the 2009 swine flu pandemic that sickened more than 60 million Americans and killed more than twelve thousand, Mount Sinai's NIH-funded Center for Research in Influenza Pathogenesis (CRIP), led by Dr. Garcia-Sastre, was highly active in, among other things, characterizing the virus, including exploring why people over sixty-five years old were less susceptible to the disease than younger people.

COVID-19 was not an influenza virus but was nonetheless one that Mount Sinai microbiologists were primed to tackle. Dr. Garcia-Sastre compared the department's pivot from flu to COVID to the ability of a highway system built for gasoline-powered vehicles to also convey a new kind of car, say, one powered by electricity. "That's an analogy, but basically, you have a way to study these viruses that can be easily adapted to study a new virus," said Dr. Garcia-Sastre, who also heads one of six NIH-funded Centers of Excellence for Influenza Research and Response to conduct research that leads to better treatments, vaccines, disease management, and pandemic prevention and preparedness. "You don't start from zero. We have research strategies that allow us to look for virus X, Y, or Z. Plug in a different virus to see how it behaves in the system, or what antivirals might work in the system."

Fundamental to the metaphorical "highway system" that scientists had built over the years were the pathways of collaboration. "At Sinai there are already bridges between clinical people, basic research people, people with different expertise," said Dr. Garcia-Sastre. "We came together very quickly."

This would be one of the most essential takeaways from a year of pandemic research: the importance of wide-ranging collaboration. "In the past, this has been developing very slowly," said Dr. Garcia-Sastre. "People in silos, academic labs doing certain research, other labs doing something different, companies working on their own—not enough interdisciplinary science to make an impact. It was clear that we needed a new paradigm in terms of finding treatments, finding vaccines."

As with the clinical effort, space—the right kind of space—was an essential piece of the emergency response. The department had long had a biosafety level-3 lab (BSL-3), which denotes bench space built to federal regulations for handling infectious material, with properly secure and isolated entrances, autoclaves to sterilize waste, and negative airflow exhausted through a HEPA filter, among other features.

Before the pandemic, about ten researchers were trained and certified to use the BSL-3 space, with three or four researchers in there at any given time. During COVID-19, the number of researchers enrolled to use the space jumped to more than 80. To accommodate the demand, a community effort that included the dean's office, engineering, the Center for Comparative Medicine and Surgery, and the Institutional Animal Care and Use Committee mobilized to rapidly convert additional space in the veterinary sciences building to the exacting standards of biosafety level-3.

"The BSL-3 labs really become a critical node in Mount Sinai's research," said Randy Albrecht, an associate professor of microbiology who serves as director of the BSL-3 facility as well as the responsible official for the school's Select Agents and Toxins program. "During COVID, all of a sudden there was a marriage of clinical and basic research, and the focal point was this BSL-3 facility, because to handle any cell culture, any clinical isolates, any patient specimens, you had to use this facility."

As did his peers on the clinical and operational front lines, Dr. Albrecht believed that the pandemic revealed the importance of looking ahead and the dangers of being guided by short-term priorities and low-margin forces, which could leave a health care system vulnerable to the next pandemic. Even if it doesn't always receive traffic that overfills a Google scheduling calendar every day with a flurry of entries (as Mount Sinai's continually did from March 2020 onward), biocontainment spaces are a necessary resource for conducting vital science in a pandemic. No way around it.

"There's always a bit of talk about, 'Do we really need them?'" Dr. Albrecht said, referring to such specialty needs as a biocontainment space. "Then something like this happens and, all of a sudden, their weight in gold comes back phenomenally. It's a testament to institutional planning to think: We need to have these kinds of facilities on site just in case."

BUILDING ON A STRONG FOUNDATION, Mount Sinai virologists' COVID breakthroughs began as early as February, before the virus had surfaced in New York, when Florian Krammer created a highly sensitive blood test that detected and measured antibodies to the new virus in the blood. This test—widely touted and widely shared—would shed light on the quality, quantity, and durability of the human immune response to SARS-CoV-2 and lead to important findings about the origins and community spread of New York City's outbreak. The test also gave Mount Sinai a tool in an early round of promising clinical interventions, convalescent plasma, at a time when there were no definitive treatments for a virus that was overwhelming the city and the Mount Sinai Health System.

Mount Sinai Micro, as its shorthand goes, developed other early insights into how the human body responded to the virus. Benjamin tenOever described an "inappropriate inflammatory response" characterized by lower than expected interferons—the body's innate antiviral defenses—combined with higher than expected cues to the inflammatory system. This shed light on how the virus might at once prompt an appropriate antibody response and trigger an overactive and dangerous inflammatory response. Microbiologist Benhur Lee created a "pseudovirus," an identical replica of the outer portion of the SARS-CoV-2 virus, enabling researchers to glean insights into antibody response without using a live virus that requires a BSL-3 lab.

On the therapeutic front, Dr. Garcia-Sastre's lab, in wide collaboration that spanned from San Francisco to Paris, investigated repurposing approved drugs as antivirals, narrowing down a vast library into a manageable subset that might target one of the hundreds of host proteins that SARS-CoV-2 interacted with. One drug, plitidepsin, which had limited clinical approval for use in multiple myeloma, was particularly effective in stopping the replication of SARS-CoV-2 when tested in human lung cells and animal models. The findings, published in *Science* in February 2021, suggested testing the small-molecule drug in clinical trials.

Led by Dr. Palese, Mount Sinai advanced a vaccine alternative designed to be cheaper and easier to produce than the big four that emerged from the pharmaceutical industry at the end of 2020. The world needed options, reasoned Dr. Palese, if it was going to tackle the extraordinary mandate to inoculate a population of nearly 8 billion. Produced in a simple chicken egg, the vaccine that the team developed used as a vector an innocuous virus called Newcastle disease virus. This methodology is similar to the adenovirus vector delivery system developed by Johnson & Johnson and AstraZeneca. Dr. Palese estimated that the Newcastle disease virus vaccine could be produced for one or two dollars per dose, vastly cheaper, he said, than the cost to produce mRNA vaccines. "We are focusing right now," he said, "on providing a vaccine approach to low- and middle-income countries," which included Vietnam, Thailand, Brazil, and Mexico. The vaccine later moved to clinical trials in those countries.

Amid nonstop COVID-19 research, Mount Sinai virologists also continued to make progress on a universal flu vaccine and advanced research with methodologies and findings providing us with salient takeaways for and beyond the COVID-19 pandemic. "These breakthroughs are certainly needed," said Dr. Garcia-Sastre. "I think this pandemic told us that we need more support to develop broad-spectrum vaccines. The same thing with antivirals and treatments. It's key. We hardly have any good treatment for viral infections, and the ones that we have, they are specific for a very specific virus. This makes it very difficult to respond fast to a pandemic if a new virus emerges."

It is by thinking more broadly than a virus-by-virus response that a global society of humans living cheek by jowl with animals can be best prepared for—or even prevent—the next pandemic.

÷

AN EARLY BREAKTHROUGH: THE QUANTITATIVE ANTIBODY TEST

'You want to help as early and as much as possible'

Nature has given us an enemy, but nature has also given us a tool to fight the enemy. Millions of people healed themselves by producing antibodies that kill the virus.

—CARLOS CORDON-CARDO, *chair of pathology*

———

IN JANUARY 2020, as the clouds of the new coronavirus gathered on the horizon, Dr. Krammer was talking with his colleague Viviana Simon about what they saw coming their way. New York City was an international crossroads, with heavy air travel to and from the rest of the world, including, of course, China. The virologists knew it was only a matter of time before people with the novel coronavirus ended up in New York. Drs. Krammer and Simon asked a central question that they, as virologists, were uniquely equipped to investigate. "So how do you find those people?" Dr. Krammer asked. "If you want to look for those infections, you need to be able to detect the virus. So we started right away assembling reagents to do that."

Dr. Krammer's area of expertise lay in understanding the body's immune response to viruses, especially the antibody response. So that was where he looked. Diagnostic tests were being developed to detect the SARS-CoV-2 RNA genome in a nasal swab, to reveal whether a person was currently infected with COVID-19. These tests were in great demand and were vital to monitor, track, and treat the virus in and out of hospitals. But Dr. Krammer got to work on a test that hunted not for the virus itself, not for signs of an active infection, but rather for a calling card that the virus had been there. That is, the antibodies the immune system musters to fight the invading virus.

Testing for antibodies could illuminate how the human body was protecting itself, as well as where and how prevalently the virus was spreading and just how deadly it was. Without knowing the "denominator" of how many people had been infected, it was impossible to know things like the infection fatality rate. The test results could also identify candidates who could donate antibody-rich blood after their recovery in the hopes that it would benefit COVID-19 patients early in their illness, before their own systems had made sufficient antibodies (see Chapter 3).

As soon as the genome was released, Dr. Krammer got to work generating the now-famous spike protein, a key characteristic of SARS-CoV-2 that enables the virus to get into cells and also gives neutralizing antibodies something to bind onto. His lab designed two versions: the full-length protein as well as a smaller piece known as the receptor-binding domain (RBD), the target of many neutralizing antibodies. The idea was to put those invaders in a dish, introduce a sample of diluted blood, and see if the antibodies in the blood react to the target. If SARS-CoV-2 antibodies are present, the reaction should produce a color change in the serum. Yellow means, yes, you have antibodies.

But the test didn't stop there. The key differentiator between Dr. Krammer's test and other antibody tests developed throughout the pandemic year lay in what happened next. Beyond the initial yellow-for-yes, the color continued to change—a deepening yellow—to reveal the *quantity* of antibodies present in the blood. That level of specificity made the test all the more valuable because it enabled researchers to answer more questions, and it formed the basis for Mount Sinai's convalescent plasma treatment program, enabling it to seek only donors who had a high level of antibodies.

To test the tests, Dr. Krammer needed positive controls— samples from patients known to have had COVID-19—as well as negative controls, patients known *not* to have had the virus. Positive samples were hard to come by at the time because Mount Sinai had not yet treated any patients who tested positive for COVID and, said Dr. Krammer, because the CDC was not sharing materials from other infected Americans, of whom there were to date very few. But the young Austrian researcher, an active member of the global scientific community, reached out to colleagues and was able to obtain samples from the University of Helsinki in Finland and the University of Melbourne in Australia.

For negative controls, he needed to reach out only as far as his colleague Dr. Simon, two floors up, who over the past three years had been collecting samples from patients with influenza and other viruses, as well as from healthy volunteers who donated blood before and after receiving vaccinations, as part of the Mount Sinai Virology Initiative she headed. In collaboration with another Mount Sinai virus-hunting initiative, the Pathogen Surveillance Program, Dr. Simon had been getting materials from infected patients in Mount Sinai hospitals, taken when clinicians performed necessary diagnostics or other health-monitoring measures. Because those samples from her program were taken before SARS-CoV-2 entered the human population, they were known to be negative.

When Dr. Krammer ran the tests, the blood known to be infected with the virus changed color. The samples that predated the virus did not. The results clearly showed the presence of antibodies to SARS-CoV-2 and answered one of the pandemic's most urgent and foundational questions: *Did infected people produce antibodies to the SARS-CoV-2 virus?* The answer, Dr. Krammer demonstrated, was yes.

From there, scientists could explore a whole host of questions, including: *Do all people who are infected mount a strong antibody response to SARS-CoV-2?* And, *How long do the antibodies—and their related protections—last?* Then there was what Dr. Krammer called the million-dollar question, *What level of antibodies is necessary to confer protection against severe illness?*

"That's the key question that I'm asking: How much antibody do we need to be protected from the virus?" he said. "It's very important for public health planning and for vaccine development."

Throughout 2020 and into 2021, Dr. Simon led an ongoing study investigating that central question. The PARIS study (Protection Associated with Rapid Immunity to SARS-CoV-2) tracked antibody levels of some 470 people, examining them every two to four weeks to get a granular look at just what the antibody levels were doing and how well the participants were protected against infection.

A seminal paper authored by Dr. Krammer, Dr. Simon, and more than two dozen collaborators described how to set up and run Mount Sinai's antibody test, essentially providing a recipe for researchers around the world to follow. An important advantage of the test, known as an enzyme-linked immunosorbent assay, or ELISA, was that it did not require the handling of highly infectious material, so researchers could develop and use it without need for a biosafety level 3 lab. The paper was posted to a preprint server in April and published in *Nature Medicine* in July.

Sharing findings widely was the scientific rule of order during the pandemic. After all, any breakthrough in getting this virus under control was a win for humanity. "That's what you do in a pandemic," Dr. Krammer said. "I did not see value in holding anything back. You want to help as early and as much as possible."

AS A RESEARCHER, Dr. Krammer couldn't use his test directly on patients. He had to translate the breakthrough—and fast—to the clinical side, which is regulated by the FDA under something called the Clinical Laboratory Improvement Amendments, or CLIA. Enter Carlos Cordon-Cardo, chair of pathology. His department connected research labs and CLIA labs, an invaluable link during the pandemic as pathologists rapidly translated new tests to clinicians scrambling for tools.

"As a research lab, we are not allowed to provide any clinical diagnostics," Dr. Simon explained on a podcast called This Week in Virology. "It would have been maddening," she said, for clinicians to know there were valid lab-developed tests but that they could not use them. "That's where the magic happened here at Mount Sinai.

Thanks to the leadership, those things became possible."

Dr. Cordon-Cardo had been consulting scientists, including the virology team, to develop a SARS-CoV-2 diagnostic test, and he immediately saw the value in the antibody test as another resource to track the disease. "The reality is that the Sinai research assay is one of the best assays available worldwide," Dr. Cordon-Cardo said. "The test that started in the research lab came into the clinical laboratories with a great deal of specificity and sensitivity—which is what you need. *Yes* or *no* in general—that's not sufficient. We want to quantify. This has been one of the most important contributions this institution has made—to have a robust assay for monitoring the disease through serology."

A number of developments happened in short order to scale the test and amplify its impact. The assay was one of the first to receive emergency use authorization from the FDA, in April, as a qualitative test, and would later be so certified (by the New York State Department of Health) as a quantitative test. In May, Mount Sinai's technology transfer office formed Kantaro Biosciences, a venture in partnership with Renalytix AI, to disseminate the antibody tests widely; as of June 2021, the test had been used more than 127,000 times on a highly diverse patient population.

"It's nice to see that there's also commercial products out there," said Dr. Krammer. "We have some of those kits that Kantaro produces here in the lab, and I like to look at them." But he is, at heart, an academic scientist and is enormously gratified by acknowledgements to his laboratory in research papers from all over the world, thanking him for the blueprint for researchers to create the ELISA test themselves. As of fall 2020, more than 250 labs nationwide and globally had developed antibody tests using his recipe, and the test had been performed on more than 68,000 people.

WHEN DR. KRAMMER'S ASSAY went up on the preprint server on April 16, 2020, COVID-19 had killed more than 145,000 people worldwide. We were still at the dawn of the pandemic, which would go on to cause more than 4.3 million deaths globally when these pages were written in August 2021, according to the Johns Hopkins Coronavirus Resource Center. There was a clamoring for information about the SARS-CoV-2 antibody response. Dr. Krammer's expertise was widely sought, not only in scientific and medical circles but also among a general public wanting to know, *How do I know if I've had the virus? If I have antibodies, how long will they last? Can I get the infection again?*

Dr. Krammer was often called upon for answers. When Anderson Cooper of CNN wanted to know more about antibody response and the possibility of reinfection, he called on Dr. Krammer. When National Public Radio wanted to know how long an immune response to SARS-CoV-2 might last, they called on Dr. Krammer. When high school students wanted to know more about how the pandemic might end and where the next one might come from, they, through an educational nonprofit called BioBus, called on Dr. Krammer, who in addition to giving them insights on the virus also shared his early dreams of becoming a scientist while growing up in a tiny Austrian village surrounded by the wonders of nature. Dr. Krammer also wrote updates, in German, to family and friends every Sunday. Those updates were translated into English, with his permission, by the Austrian website Metropole and posted each week to a wider audience. On Twitter, where he has 210,000 followers, he did a 138-tweet-long tweetorial explaining vaccines.

As time passed, Mount Sinai researchers got a clearer picture of how long antibodies appeared to last, including a finding in July that the majority of people who had COVID, even a mild case, mounted a robust antibody response that remained stable for at least three months. Preprinted in July, and in the *Lancet Microbe* in September, the study was led by Ania Wajnberg, an internal medicine doctor who was head of Mount Sinai's outpatient ambulatory practices and oversaw the clinical implementation of the health system's convalescent plasma program.

Another study led by Dr. Wajnberg, published in *Science* in December (preprinted October), found that antibody titers are relatively stable for at least five months, and that most people infected with mild-to-moderate COVID-19 experience robust immunoglobulin G antibody responses against the viral spike protein. The study was based on 30,082 individuals who, when screened as potential convalescent plasma donors, tested positive for antibodies.

One of the key themes that Dr. Krammer drew from his and his colleagues' findings was that when it came to antibody response, SARS-CoV-2 behaved, in the main, like a coronavirus. Presenting to an institution-wide research event in November, Dr. Krammer enumerated the following conclusions:

- *Humans induce solid antibody responses to SARS-CoV-2, even after mild infection*
- *Antibodies binding to the spike protein correlate with neutralization*
- *The antibody response looks normal for a respiratory virus:*
  - *Initial strong increase driven by plasmablast*
  - *Decline over time after that (IgG long half life=21 days)*
  - *Seem to stabilize at a certain level (driven by long-lived plasma cells)*

When asked in an interview whether he felt that he was hunting down a medical mystery, he answered, "I think what we learned more and more is that this virus behaves like a coronavirus. The problem is that human coronaviruses were hard to study because nobody was interested in them. Now there's a lot of data that basically confirms things we knew before. We found also new things that will probably lead to discoveries with the common cold coronaviruses, as well. So I don't really see this as a medical mystery."

There were plenty of biomedical mysteries still to be solved about how to treat the virus, what it did to the lungs and to the cardiovascular and immune systems, COVID's effect on children, the multifarious debilitation of lingering disease, and many other troubling questions. But what Dr. Krammer's lab came to discover about SARS-CoV-2 seroconversion—or, the body's production of antibodies following infection—was a pivotal early finding in a pandemic that would go on to confound so many other provinces of science and medicine.

✢

TRACKING THE VIRUS'S PATH
'It's a global phenomenon'

When a virus makes new copies of itself, small mistakes can be introduced in its genome, much like you can make typos when copying a text. These small mistakes leave a genetic fingerprint that we can trace to understand the evolutionary history of the virus. That's, in a nutshell, the genetic analysis of the viral genome and the story that that tells us about how it has spread and changed over time.
—HONORATUS VAN BAKEL, *director, Pathogen Surveillance Program*

———

ONCE MOUNT SINAI received its first patient suspected to have COVID-19 on February 29, virologists, genomic scientists, and clinicians would team up to track the fingerprints and footprints of SARS-CoV-2 in New York City. They would come to learn how long the virus had been circulating in the city and the route by which the virus came ashore, which would prove to be other than what politicians and policymakers had taken early action against.

With patients starting to surge and in-house diagnostic testing getting the go-ahead, Viviana Simon, along with colleagues Honoratus (Harm) Van Bakel and Emilia Mia Sordillo, collected more and more clinical specimens left over from the health system's diagnostic nasal swabs. A team of researchers isolated the virus from Mount Sinai's first confirmed COVID-19 patient and sequenced its genome. "Within a week, we had the sequence of the genome to be shared," said Dr. Simon. "And when I say we, I truly mean *we*."

She described a "gigantic collaboration" that spanned her lab, as well as those of Dr. Sordillo, director of clinical microbiology laboratories, and Dr. Van Bakel, one of the codirectors of the Mount Sinai Pathogen Surveillance Program. "We're really joined at the hip," said Dr. Van Bakel, who is a genetic and genomic scientist.

Some of the work, such as the hands-on processing of samples, happened in clinical microbiology and research labs, including biosafety level 2 and level 3 labs. Scientists also got to work analyzing data on the computer. "Once we generated the sequencing data, we had to establish new assembly, genome comparison, and phylogenetic analysis pipelines for a novel virus that had just emerged," outlined Dr. Van Bakel. For the study of a completely novel virus, he found himself drawing on lessons learned and infrastructure established for the Mount Sinai Pathogen Surveillance Program.

The Pathogen Surveillance Program was started in 2014 to bring genomics and genome sequencing into the clinical microbiology lab in order to track pathogens in Mount Sinai's patient population. Genomic sequencing—deciphering the exact DNA code at work—gave scientists a powerful tool to see how the virus, case by case, was changing over time and where outbreaks were occurring.

"We can map the genomes of pathogens just like we do for humans, and that gives us some information about how they spread," said Dr. Van Bakel. "So, okay, if you have a cluster of cases in a particular location in the Mount Sinai Health System, we can say whether or not they're related to each other and whether or not there may be some local outbreak happening. We can also look for resistant and novel variants."

Typical pathogens in the program's sights had included bacterial infections such as methicillin-resistant *Staphylococcus aureus* (MRSA) and *Clostridium difficile*. The program also examined seasonal flu virus, working alongside Mount Sinai's prodigious influenza research teams and the Mount Sinai Virology Initiative. Dr. Van Bakel pointed to an outbreak of seasonal flu a year earlier, in 2019, that sickened more than 90 patients and health care workers, which the Pathogen Surveillance Program had traced to learn how the outbreak started and how it spread.

"We can help hospital epidemiologists lock down outbreaks before they happen or become too large to control," explained Dr. Simon. "We retooled our program from respiratory viruses in general, and flu in specific, to become fully focused on SARS-CoV-2."

"Fully focused on SARS-CoV-2" cannot be overstated. In the two weeks after Mount Sinai got the go-ahead to COVID-test in-house on March 17, the health system saw as many positive COVID cases as it would normally see positive flu cases during an entire year.

While the name sounds like something out of a science fiction movie, the Pathogen Surveillance Program's real-world tools and expertise in phylogenetic analysis had never been more in demand. The questions it was built to answer were urgent matters in a city under siege: *Where in the world had New York's COVID-19 pathogen come from, and how was it spreading through the city?* The United States had enacted a series of travel restrictions, starting with flights from China, yet the virus had still arrived—and, as would soon be revealed, in numbers that throughout most of 2020 were the highest in the world.

The team quickly sequenced virus from the first two patients to test positive in the Mount Sinai Health System—the patient who had returned from Iran and was seen at the Mount Sinai Hospital February 29 and Rodrigo Saval, the Chilean whose epic COVID journey began at Mount Sinai West on March 7, following a trip to Europe.

"What we found there was expected," said Dr. Van Bakel. "We had one traveler with a Middle Eastern travel history, and we found a viral genome that clustered with other Middle Eastern cases. We had another traveler with a European travel history, which clustered with European cases."

Beyond that, he said, scientists weren't quite sure what they'd find when they sampled subsequent patients receiving care at Mount Sinai. "With this big surge we saw in mid-March, we weren't sure whether we would see that the introduction to New York City was related to travelers from China or from other regions in the world," said Dr. Van Bakel.

A wide-ranging team from the Icahn Institute for Data Science and Genomic Technology, the Global Health and Emerging Pathogens Institute, and the departments of microbiology, pathology, and genetics and genomic sciences sequenced the SARS-CoV-2 genomes obtained from 84 out of the 800-plus confirmed COVID-19 cases across the Mount Sinai Health System at the time, February 29 to March 18. The cases were drawn from 21 New York City neighborhoods across four boroughs—Manhattan, Bronx, Queens, and Brooklyn— as well as two towns in neighboring Westchester County. The team then analyzed these sequences together with 2,363 publicly available SARS-CoV-2 genomes from around the world to determine the most likely origin of the virus strains infecting Mount Sinai patients, a microcosm of New York City.

"What we found is that the overwhelming majority of the introduction of the virus here in the city did not come directly from China, but rather came indirectly from travelers from Europe," said Dr. Van Bakel, whose findings were posted online in April—to a flurry of media attention—and later published in *Science*. "It made a stopover in Europe, and the cases that we saw here in New York City were really introduced by travelers from Europe."

Further, the study estimated that SARS-CoV-2 was first introduced in New York in early February—weeks before the first COVID-19 patient in New York State walked through Mount Sinai's doors.

The takeaway? "It's a global phenomenon," said Dr. Van Bakel. "You can't focus on one area. In the beginning, there was, 'Okay, we need to shut down travel from China. We need to limit travel from *here* and *here*.' But as those efforts were underway, we were actually already starting to see cases coming in through travelers from Europe. You need to have a holistic approach."

In addition, the researchers found related viruses clustered among patients living in different neighborhoods across the city, suggesting community transmission was already underway in New York in early March.

The timeline of introduction to New York would be bolstered by a subsequent study, this time using Dr. Krammer's ELISA antibody test to track COVID-19 footprints in more than 10,000 plasma samples taken from the beginning of February to July. The samples were taken from patients coming to the Mount Sinai Hospital for non-COVID-related care, including emergency and routine care. The first samples to show antibodies in the blood were taken during the week of February 23, which would mean the virus had been contracted even earlier.

The researchers also found that by late May, about 20 percent of the plasma samples were seropositive, meaning they contained antibodies. In other words, about 20 percent of New Yorkers—some 1.7 million people—may well have had COVID-19 by the time the first devastating wave was over.

In addition, now that they knew the denominator—that is, how many people had been infected—researchers could determine that infection fatality rate. About 1 percent, they found, which is ten times more deadly than seasonal flu.

The fact that COVID was scything through New York before it ever surfaced in hospitals revealed the need to test vastly more than the United States had in the early weeks and months of the pandemic. "If you don't have large-scale screening ability to detect the virus, it will stay under the radar," said Dr. Van Bakel. "You really need to have a much broader testing initiative so that you can find it in the community."

STUDYING 'A DISEASE OF MULTIPLE DISEASES'

'Why were some people dying and some people not?'

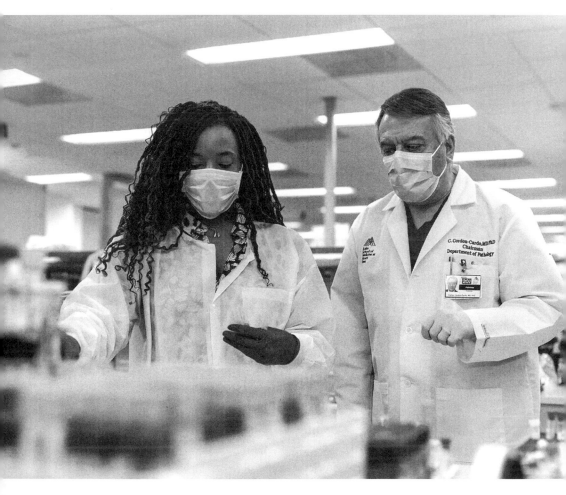

Pathologist Carlos Cordon-Cardo, above with technician Nina Dominic, investigated what COVID-19 did to the body and translated research findings to the clinic.

EARLY IN THE SARS-COV-2 OUTBREAK, Mount Sinai virologists discovered that the novel coronavirus prompted a fairly typical production of antibodies. But—as clinicians were seeing on the front lines—the disease sent other systems into chaos. This was a respiratory disease with cardiovascular implications and an immune dysregulation that begged for further study. Some patients got severely or fatally ill, while others navigated the disease with no symptoms. The destruction seemed as capricious as it was comprehensive.

COVID-19 disproportionately affected the vulnerable, the elderly, the chronically ill, people of color, while seeming to largely spare children—but not always. SARS-CoV-2 was a virus that demanded to be explored both in its rules and in its apparent exceptions to those rules. Just when science and medicine seemed to have a handle on a certain aspect of the disease, another frightening wrinkle would unfold and open up new questions.

Chief pathologist Carlos Cordon-Cardo called COVID-19 "a disease of multiple diseases." Its rampant heterogeneity drew an array of Mount Sinai scientists to the SARS-CoV-2 research enterprise, not only virologists but immunologists, oncologists, cardiovascular physicians and scientists, radiologists, and the all-important pathologists to translate breakthroughs in the lab to tools in the clinic and lessons from autopsies to practice in patients. Mount Sinai also mobilized more than a hundred young researchers to build the COVID-19 Biobank, a real-time trove to inform scientists now and into the future.

✣

PATHOLOGY: WHAT THE DEAD CAN TEACH THE LIVING

'The autopsy opened our eyes big-time'

Most patients know their pediatrician, general practitioner, surgeon, oncologist. But nobody knows the pathologist—or the critical role we play at every juncture of life. From the moment you're born and

have your newborn screening to when your clinician runs lab tests to understand why you feel unlike yourself, we are there for you. It is not "the lab" that brings you and your clinicians that critical information or helps guide the hand of your surgeon. It is, behind the microscope, a large team of devoted pathologists and technical staff. We see you from the moment you are born to when the soul departs your body.

—CARLOS CORDON-CARDO, *chair of pathology*

———

MARCH 1, 2020—When Mount Sinai confirmed the state's first COVID-positive patient, Carlos Cordon-Cardo immediately called the chief medical officer of the City of New York, Barbara Sampson. Envisioning what was coming and his health system's role in both caring for the sick and advancing a scientific understanding of the disease, he wanted to share key developments that he and his colleague, Mary Fowkes, director of Mount Sinai's autopsy service, were planning. That included performing autopsies on patients who succumbed to COVID-19, as well as ordering six refrigerator trucks, just in case the death toll warranted it.

Within weeks, the refrigerator trucks were packed, as people were falling sick and dying in unfathomable numbers across the health system, as they were across other New York City hospitals. Funeral homes were overwhelmed, delaying burials and later closing, as did cemeteries. And Mount Sinai pathologists, tragically, had an unprecedented number of deceased patients whose bodies contained important clues to the novel virus that was ravaging New York.

"We have worked very hard to make sure you have the best chance to be cured, with the best quality of life and all of the dignity that you deserve," said Dr. Cordon-Cardo, speaking with the cadence of a storyteller to an imaginary patient on a typical journey of care. "And if something goes wrong, I'm going to take that body, and I'm going to treat it with the dignity it deserves. And if the final decision of the family or the person before dying is to donate the body to us to further understand, this is the ultimate act of kindness you can give to society." He described an invocation passed through generations of pathologists at the time of autopsy: *Can you help us understand*

what happened to you?

"What was the biology of this disease, why were people dying?" Dr. Cordon-Cardo asked, continuing to unspool the story. "What was the physiology, the understanding of the disease and the extent of organ damage? For that we needed autopsies—and we did more COVID-19 autopsies than most any academic department of pathology during the early pandemic. That allowed us to understand that this was not only a respiratory disease. This was a complex disease of multiple phases and affecting many organs."

One of Mount Sinai pathology's most important contributions to the science of COVID-19 and what it did to the body came out of a series of autopsies performed in New York's first pandemic wave. Pathologists would find that, in addition to being a respiratory disease, SARS-CoV-2 also attacked the endothelial cells lining the blood vessels, weakening them and rendering the blood prone to clotting. Clinicians on the floors were asking similar questions and having similar insights into hypercoagulability. Together, these insights informed Mount Sinai's rapidly deployed anticoagulation protocol (described in Chapter 3), which would soon become standard practice worldwide for COVID-19 patients.

Pathology also played an instrumental role from the very beginning of the pandemic in translating from the laboratory to the clinical floor tests such as Dr. Krammer's ELISA assay to test for antibodies and Mount Sinai's molecular-based COVID diagnostic test.

Pathology, after all, is used to putting clinical medicine under a microscope.

For Dr. Cordon-Cardo, the love of a microscope has been with him since he asked for one for his tenth birthday (rather than the piano his family wanted to get him). "Since then, I knew that my passion was what I'm doing now, every day," said Dr. Cordon-Cardo, his baritone voice resonating with that passion. Today, working at his office and in the labs of one of the most prestigious academic medical centers in the world, he is filled with the same sense of inspiration and curiosity, he says, that he experienced as a boy in the lab he fashioned in the basement of his family's Barcelona home.

THE OVERRIDING COMPLAINT sending people to the hospital during the COVID-19 outbreak was shortness of breath. But patients also displayed a diverse array of symptoms that at first puzzled clinicians and researchers. Dr. Cordon-Cardo cited a patient with, yes, trouble breathing, but also nightmares and night sweats. There were memory lapses, leaving, for example, an English teacher unable to spell. There was neuropsychiatric symptomology, Dr. Cordon-Cardo said, and an increase in strokes, even among the young and previously healthy.

"What are we missing here?" the pathologists were asking.

They would begin to find answers in the autopsies.

Performing an autopsy in the best of times is a meticulous endeavor, incising with the skill of a surgeon, investigating with the acuity of a detective. During COVID, there were many additional challenges, including obtaining consent over the phone from families who were in quarantine and had been separated from their loved ones during death; the need to wear the highest level of protective equipment, a PAPR, or powered air-purifying respirator, an astronaut-like full-body suit, hood, and mask that uses a filtered air system; and sheer fear of the virus's spread. Wearing the "space suit" and leading the autopsies in the basement of the Mount Sinai Hospital was pathologist Mary Fowkes, who directed Mount Sinai's autopsy service.

"I've always thought that autopsies were important, but then when COVID hit, it just hit me so hard how important they can be," she told Mount Sinai's podcast, Real, Smart People. "I was one of four pathologists here at Mount Sinai that were willing to volunteer to do the COVID autopsies, despite the risk." So aware was she of the risk that she didn't tell her children she was performing autopsies—but her cover was blown when a colleague posted a picture of her in full PAPR.

"Because we don't know anything about this disease, an autopsy is the most useful, because it will help us determine how the virus is actually making people sick," she told CBS's 60 Minutes.

Dr. Cordon-Cardo tells the story of an early patient on whom the team performed an autopsy. He'd come in with a temperature of about ninety-nine degrees, not really a fever. Upon entry to the hospital, he immediately showed signs of severe inflammation, atrial fibrillation, then asystole, a fatal cardiac arrest.

This was no straightforward respiratory illness.

"The autopsy opened our eyes big-time," said Dr. Cordon-Cardo. "In the brain we saw all of these hemorrhages and thromboembolisms that didn't allow the blood to move to the blood vessels because they were occluded."

Mount Sinai pathologists went on to perform more than 100 autopsies during the first wave, from March 20 to June 23, and published studies that would impact how scientists and clinicians would come to understand the multifarious disease and explore potential treatments. While almost all the autopsies revealed damage consistent with respiratory disease, it was the myriad other damages that were perhaps more revelatory.

"Our autopsy series of COVID-19-positive patients reveals that this disease, often conceptualized as a primarily respiratory viral illness, has widespread effects in the body including hypercoagulability, a hyperinflammatory state, and endothelial dysfunction," said the paper analyzing the findings, published in *Modern Pathology* in April 2021 (with a remarkable 54 authors), after having been preprinted much earlier, in May 2020, with the result of 67 autopsies. "Targeting of these multisystemic pathways could lead to new treatment avenues as well as combination therapies against SARS-CoV-2 infection."

"It's a disease of multiple diseases," Dr. Cordon-Cardo explained, "which we have to compare to complex diseases such as cancer. COVID-19 starts in the nose, but it goes into your lungs, into your liver, into your brain." SARS-CoV-2 *metastasized*, he noted, as cancer can do. And he pointed to the word's Greek etymology, meaning "moving away from origin." "That was what SARS-CoV-2 achieved," he said, "moving through blood vessels from the nose to distant organs, such as the brain."

The blood clotting that was emerging as a dangerous symptom of COVID-19 was at the center of the autopsy findings. The study suggested that the virus causes damage to the endothelial cells, the thin layer of cells that line the blood vessels, and that weakening underlies the clotting abnormalities. Pathologists found blood clots throughout the body but, importantly, found pulmonary emboli as well as blood clots in the brain causing both small and large strokes. In 17 of the 58 brains they evaluated, pathologists found "widespread presence of microthrombi," or tiny blood clots, as Dr. Fowkes and her autopsy team described.

Researchers also noticed a dropping off of pulmonary emboli after April 9, when Mount Sinai implemented a standardized anticoagulation protocol throughout its hospitals (see Chapter 3). This could mean, the study posited, that the course of blood-thinners patients were given contributed to the decline in pulmonary embolism as a cause of death in Mount Sinai's patients. The researchers were quick to note, however, that they autopsied only a fraction of the system's patients, and that they did not control for other factors, which certainly could have played a role.

Pathologists also saw evidence of elevated cytokines, which are small proteins that regulate immunity. Those were signs of the hyperinflammatory state, the immune system's overactive response to the virus, which clinicians had flagged as a dangerous complication in their patients. This finding added to a growing body of evidence that was prompting Mount Sinai immunologists to explore this inflammation, what was causing it, how to diagnose it early, and how to treat it (which we will explore in depth in the next chapter).

The pandemic, said Dr. Fowkes, "highlighted the importance of autopsies, especially in situations where the disease is new or newly emerging, where we don't entirely understand how it is causing symptoms and resulting in death. It's the gold standard for understanding what a disease is doing."

IN NOVEMBER, Dr. Fowkes died suddenly of a heart attack at her home (her autopsy, Dr. Cordon-Cardo noted, revealed no presence of COVID). Dr. Cordon-Cardo and many of her colleagues praised her for her role in deepening medicine's understanding of the pandemic and informing clinical care, beginning at Mount Sinai and having ripple effects across the world. At the time of her death, she was exploring what autopsies might reveal about the causes of the highly multifarious, multi-organ post-acute COVID syndrome, or PACS.

There were seeds of PACS findings, as well, in the initial Mount Sinai autopsy study. The authors, including Drs. Fowkes and Cordon-Cardo, suggested that the clotting in blood vessels throughout the brain might help explain neurological changes such as confusion and brain fog in COVID patients, as well as what the paper called "the still ill-defined post-COVID neurological sequelae beginning to emerge."

Dr. Cordon-Cardo was determined to press autopsies into service to explore post-acute COVID. He enlisted the New York City chief medical examiner and other pathology groups across the state to begin investigating what he called "unnatural deaths"—suicides, accidents, sudden unexplained deaths, particularly in younger people—and to see if the deceased showed evidence of having had COVID-19. Any correlations found here could provide vital clues to how the lingering illness affected a body, a life, a family, and a community.

⁙

IMMUNOLOGY: FINDING THE BALANCE
'Immunologists became an extremely important part of the story'

You cannot treat what you don't understand. It's a very important principle in medicine. You can treat the symptoms, yes, but if you don't stop what's causing the symptoms, you're not going to stop the disease. Scientists came together to go to the root of what was causing this disease.

—MIRIAM MERAD, *director of Mount Sinai's Precision Immunology Institute*

MIRIAM MERAD BEGAN her career as an oncologist hoping she could practice both her passions equally—treating patients and driving science. But her early days as a busy practicing clinician left too little time for research. So she shifted her focus. "I realized I was treating the symptoms, but I was not understanding really how this cancer was progressing," said Dr. Merad, whose passion for her work stands out even in a community of devoted and zealous scientists. "So at some point I made the decision to focus on the science, even if it broke my heart to do it. I come from a big family of scientists, and clinical care was very much what I was raised with and had wanted to do since I was a little child."

Research is driven by questions. Every answer begets a new series of questions. With COVID-19, the first question an immunologist might ask is: *Could the body even mount an immune response to SARS-CoV-2?* That question, noted Dr. Merad, was answered in February by her Mount Sinai colleague a couple of buildings over. With his ELISA assay showing the presence of antibodies, Florian Krammer had found that the body does produce an immune response to SARS-CoV-2, and it appeared to be robust.

Further confirmation came from the earliest Mount Sinai autopsies, which found that some patients who succumbed to the disease had little or no virus left in the body. "The immune system was able to completely get rid of the virus, and yet the patients continue to get worse," noted Dr. Merad. The problem for many of the sickest patients, it turned out, was not that the immune system failed to produce a response but that the immune response was for some reason too robust, had grown out of control.

The next overarching question was *why?*

"This is where immunologists became an extremely important part of the story, because this is what we do—study immune response to threat," said Dr. Merad, who, among other groundbreaking findings in the past, has identified fundamental characteristics of macrophages, large specialized white blood cells, and made important connections to cancer progression and response to treatment, and to inflammatory bowel disease.

Harnessing the immune system—in the right way at the right time for the right patient—is one of the most salient therapeutic pursuits in medicine today, including the elegant art and precise science of immunotherapy to treat cancer. Although they are very different illnesses, there were some important similarities between COVID and cancer. Both diseases had a high degree of heterogeneity—the illness manifesting in many different ways in different patients—and both suggested an opportunity to modulate the immune system in order to regulate the disease. Dr. Merad and her team, including researchers Sacha Gnjatic and Thomas Marron, drew on vast oncology expertise and resources to make some important findings in COVID-19.

"Cancer immunotherapy researchers were quite prepared to address this type of medical problem," said Dr. Merad. "We think about heterogeneity all the time, trying to understand why some cancer patients respond to immunotherapy and why some do not respond."

For their investigation, Mount Sinai immunologists pivoted off an existing platform used for cancer patients. Patients with multiple myeloma can be treated with immunotherapies called CAR T-cells, a certain immune cell introduced into their system to fight the blood borne cancer. The T-cells' response to the cancer can, in some cases, be so rapid that it triggers overwhelming inflammation—the so called cytokine release storm, similar to what COVID patients experienced—which can be deadly if left untreated. But Mount Sinai immunologists had developed a rapid test to measure cytokine levels after treatment for multiple myeloma patients and enable doctors to act quickly with counteractive therapies if necessary.

In early March, the immunologists worked with pathologists to bring the rapid multiplex cytokine assay directly to the COVID wards to give clinicians there an additional window into a patient's condition. Clinicians were already looking at other biomarkers to better understand a patient's condition and inform treatment, such as blood oxygen levels to determine if a patient needed supplemental oxygen and D-dimer levels that indicated blood-clotting potential. "All these were being looked at, and we added cytokines onto that assessment of the patient," explained Sacha Gnjatic, a tumor immunologist who pivoted his work to COVID immune research during the pandemic. "Thanks to the pathology department, our test became authorized for clinical use by the New York State Department of Health. That allowed us to test a huge number of patients in a very rapid amount of time by just having the clinicians who see these patients order the test in Epic," which is Mount Sinai's electronic health record.

Talk about bench to bedside. "That changed completely the way that we typically do research, where you go get the samples and bring everything to the laboratory," said Dr. Gnjatic. "Now, we just had it ordered automatically through the electronic health record."

The scientists measured four cytokines, individual strains of the Gordian knot that is the immune system. These four—interleukin (IL)-6, IL-8, tumor necrosis factor (TNF)-α, and IL-1β—were known to be involved in inflammation, and their measurement could give clinicians and scientists a window into how their levels correlated with disease severity. Might an elevated IL-6 or TNF be a predictor of severe illness or even death? And could these insights help scientists home in on targeted treatments?

One therapeutic option to block inflammation had begun to take shape on clinical floors, including those at Mount Sinai. In earlier pages, you read about Joseph Mathew deciding to treat patient Rodrigo Saval with a corticosteroid called dexamethasone, which appeared to stabilize Mr. Saval's condition. Dexamethasone is an anti-inflammatory and immunosuppressant used to treat a variety of conditions and was shown to benefit certain COVID patients by taming their hyperinflammatory response.

But, Dr. Merad cautioned, the use of steroids to treat COVID-19 involved a trick of timing, because the treatment blocks both the good and the bad immune responses. Give the steroid too early in the disease, Mount Sinai doctors found, and it was detrimental, since it blocked the antiviral immune response and prevented the production of antibodies to fight the disease. The steroid was beneficial only once the disease had become advanced and a patient was critically ill because then the drug blocks the pathogenic inflammation.

There had to be a better way, therapy that could be given earlier, that didn't blunt the entire inflammatory response but was more targeted. "We want to do much better than dexamethasone," said Dr. Merad. "We want to give something that targets the bad inflammation without targeting the beneficial one, so that we can start it early in the disease—and not wait until patients are critically ill. We want to be much smarter in blocking particular pathways that will be very damaging but will have no effect on antiviral immunity."

Early guidance came as a result of the assay to measure cytokine signatures, which the team put in place in March on the floors of the hospital. After testing 1,484 patients between March 20 and early June and adjusting for a number of clinical factors, the researchers found that "IL-6 and TNF-α [blood] serum levels remained independent and significant predictors of disease severity and death," according to the study, published in *Nature Medicine* in August 2020. "We propose that serum IL-6 and TNF-α levels should be considered in the management and treatment of patients with COVID-19 to stratify prospective clinical trials, guide resource allocation and inform therapeutic options."

IL-6 and TNF were of particular interest because there are existing drugs that can act on them, and trials were proceeding apace throughout 2020 and into 2021. "This is what we are still working on, trying to identify with the pathway the beneficial versus the damaging," said Dr. Merad. "That's a big, big, big question for us right now."

The ups and downs of IL-6 clinical trials are illustrative of pandemic research and elusive answers, with some patients seeming to benefit and others not, with some clinical trials yielding successful results, others not, and still others inconclusive. These were the necessary trials—and tribulations—of science. Mount Sinai joined pharmaceutical company Regeneron's randomized controlled trial for an IL-6 blockade early in the pandemic's first wave, with great hope. But in September, a press release of the phase-three results of the trial showed that the drug was no better than the placebo.

From the floors of the hospital, Judith Aberg, chief of infectious diseases for the health system, was disappointed. "In the beginning, there was so much promise for that drug," said Dr. Aberg, who was principal investigator of multiple COVID-19 prevention and treatment trials. "Even for myself. I had one patient that got better, which was all coincidental, probably. I'm blinded, so I don't know what anybody received. But then it became apparent that nobody was really responding. It was like giving a massive dose of Tylenol. It'll get rid of your fever, but it doesn't alleviate whatever the underlying cause is."

Subsequently, doctors learned that the drug, sarilumab, and other immune-modulating medications appear to have benefit only when given with dexamethasone.

A number of IL-6 blockade trials, including from Regeneron and Roche, yielded disappointing results in 2020. But Dr. Merad still held out hope—and pointed to a later trial, a larger trial out of the United Kingdom, which showed beneficial results with IL-6 blockade by tocilizumab. In February 2021, the Randomised Evaluation of COVID-19 Therapy, or RECOVERY trial, showed that tocilizumab, when co-administered with steroids, improved survival in severely ill, hospitalized patients, among other benefits.

As these pages went to press, Dr. Merad was eagerly awaiting the results of TNF trials, poised on that knife's edge of science's promise. "I am quite excited about TNF blockades now being tried, but, see, there's a little bit of reality check here and also knowledge that you have to have about the clinical research enterprise," she said. Rigorous trials, carefully structured and precisely stratified, take time. Clinicians in the midst of treating patients do not have the luxury of time—and this is where scientists play a vital role.

Science is a series of questions. And after almost a year and a half of looking at COVID data every day, Dr. Merad was still asking one of the big questions she had been asking from the start: *Why does the immune system not understand that it needs to stop?* This is called resolution of inflammation, and figuring it out for COVID-19 would have import and impact well beyond the pandemic. Resolution of inflammation—or, more accurately, its failure—is at the heart of many diseases and conditions. Inflammatory bowel disease, rheumatoid arthritis, multiple sclerosis, and, Dr. Merad believes, aging: "All these conditions where inflammation persists and we cannot stop it."

"WILL LIFE EVER go back to normal?" Dr. Merad was asked by *New York Times* reporter Apoorva Mandavilli in a conversation at New York's 92nd Street Y held on March 16, 2021, in a distinctly different climate than the devastation of a year earlier. At that time, vaccinations were well underway in the United States and cases were dropping (although that was not so everywhere in the world, nor would it remain the case even in the United States, as the Delta variant took hold later in 2021).

"I'm an optimist because I'm an immunologist," Dr. Merad said. "My answer is that immune systems always win. So, yes, I think we will go back to normal."

⁜

BUILDING A BIOBANK:
SLEUTHING SECRETS IN THE BLOOD

'If we could understand it, maybe we could help solve it'

What the hell happened here? Why were some people dying and some people not? We now have the resource to be able to investigate those questions. It would have been a real tragedy if we didn't do this, and two years from now we were sitting here saying, 'I wish we'd sampled the people with COVID when they were really sick, so we could study what happened.'

—ALEXANDER CHARNEY, *neuroscientist, co-leader of COVID-19 Biobank*

IMMUNOLOGISTS WERE LEARNING a lot from the cytokine assay they'd translated to the clinical floor in the first weeks of the surge. But to more deeply understand the complexity of how COVID-19 affected the immune and other systems' responses over time, they and colleagues across Mount Sinai needed a *prospective* collection, a large set of samples taken from a wide variety of patients, taken at multiple time intervals, from initial hospitalization to discharge, if it came, and ideally to recovery. There were now hundreds of patients in Mount Sinai hospitals, and Miriam Merad knew that their blood and tissue contained secrets of the disease's pathophysiology and clues to potential therapies.

And she knew her institution. Mount Sinai prided itself on learning from the enormous and diverse population it cared for, in a mutually beneficial relationship that then drives scientific advancements directly to patients. Further, Dr. Merad knew her dean and his commitment to science in the service of patients.

So she went into Dean Dennis Charney's office to discuss collecting clinical samples and building what would become an invaluable biomedical resource.

"We need to see big," she said.

"I remember vividly what he said," she recalled. "He answered, 'The limit is the sky. You go as big as you want. I'll find the money.'"

Thus began a dramatic and high-impact mobilization across the research and clinical enterprises to help scientists and physicians answer vital questions about the human body's response to and potential therapies for COVID-19, for the post-acute form of the illness, and even for myriad other diseases that implicate the immune system.

"What is happening in the immune system that leads some people to die and some people to be fine?" asked Alexander Charney, a psychiatrist, geneticist, and neuroscientist (and Dennis Charney's son) who joined Dr. Merad in spearheading the COVID-19 Biobank collection. "It's one thing to study the virus in a [Petri] dish. It's another thing to study cells from blood that's sampled every day from 800 people during the height of their infection, and regularly after that as they're getting treated and getting better or getting worse—then seeing what happened in the samples as some people got worse versus others as they got better. *Were certain genes activated, turned on or turned off? Were certain proteins up or down?"*

To get answers, scientists would need to interrogate a dynamic resource like the one Mount Sinai began formally collecting on March 31, when there were 1,265 COVID patients across its hospitals. It would take a lot of data to yield answers. If any good could come out of Mount Sinai's rapidly mounting COVID patient census, maybe it would be the sheer volume of information researchers could glean from patients in order to ultimately heal them.

"Can we identify the pathway to hit so that we can reduce these patient casualties? That was the mandate," said Dr. Merad, who headed the Human Immune Monitoring Center, which would be analyzing the samples.

Compared to previous collections, for clinical trials, this one was on a whole new order of magnitude. Typically, said Dr. Merad, researchers collect samples from a few patients a week in any given clinical trial. In the first 49 days of the COVID-19 Biobank, researchers collected and banked samples from more than 500 patients, taken at multiple time points. The project continued even as the surge receded, eventually banking samples from more than 800 COVID patients. These were taken from a wide array of patients, mostly adults but also children. Most patients recovered and were discharged home after an average of about two weeks. Some died of the disease, and their samples, including organs post-autopsy, provided an invaluable window into the disease's most lethal iterations. Some would go on to suffer from lingering symptoms, so-called long-haulers whose sequelae remain even well after the acute phase of the disease. Samples were also taken from non-COVID patients, because every experiment needs a set of matched controls.

Mindful of the laborious process of enrolling people in a human research study—and mindful that COVID demanded a new, exigent way of operating—Alex Charney and Miriam Merad began to envision just what they would need. "If you want to collect samples from just about every person who's admitted for COVID in the middle of a pandemic, you're going to need an army of research coordinators," said Dr. Alex Charney. "Which we had. All these research coordinators whose [non-COVID] projects had been shut down were now just sitting at home doing nothing. So we put it together: *All right, let's build a big army of research staff that are going to execute every component of this giant process of getting biospecimens for COVID research.*"

THE DAY BEGAN EARLY, 5 or 6 a.m. for the morning shift, in a giant relay that would become, for many of the young redeployed researchers, the mission of a lifetime. Over the course of the long, long day, more than a hundred biobankers were broken into teams to screen electronic medical records, obtain consent from patients or families, assemble collection kits to deliver to hospital floors, reach out to nurses, transport specimens from hospital to lab, and process and eventually "bank" the samples.

The first step in the relay involved members of the screening team perusing the health system's electronic medical records for patients who'd just come into the hospital, at first the Mount Sinai Hospital adjacent to the medical school and, later, to the other uptown hospitals, Mount Sinai West and Mount Sinai Morningside. With input from clinicians, the team selected potential participants, COVID and non-COVID patients, across a wide range of eligibility requirements. Their blood would be sampled at regular intervals, beginning on Day 1, Day 3, and so on, depending on how long they were in the hospital.

Meanwhile, on the fifth floor of the largely empty Hess Building, the assembly team packed Vacutainers into biohazard bags, creating kits that would soon go to the floors for the collection process. "These assembly lines were something to behold," Alex Charney marveled. "At any given time, there were a hundred hospitalized patients in the study, and we had three different hospitals going. That's lots of tubes and bags. It was pretty impressive how these young researchers just put together this system. No one told them how to do it."

Biobank "runners" fanned out across the floors of the hospitals to pick up fresh samples each day and drop off empty kits for the next draw. During one young runner's first trip to the hospital floor, she and her team saw a patient code, receive CPR, then die, behind transparent ICU doors. "These are kids who'd never spent time on a hospital unit before," said Dr. Charney, who served as a sounding board and guide to the young researchers. "They'd certainly never seen someone die right in front of their eyes."

Project leader Nicole Simons talked with the team member for whom this was Day 1 on the job, and even referred her to one of the psychiatrists on the team. "She told me how much it helped knowing people were there to support her and that other people were feeling what she was feeling," Ms. Simons recalled.

Outreach to clinicians, especially nurses, was critical to the project's success, and eventually members of the biobank team joined in the nurses' daily huddle. The researchers were acutely aware of the pressure clinicians were under on the hospital floors and arranged for samples to be collected when nurses did their regular morning blood draws. Then, instead of sending the blood to the clinical labs for analysis, the clinicians would simply leave the samples for the biobank runners to pick up. "We emphasized that we were not giving patients an extra needle stick," said Ms. Simons.

To make sure the runners were easy to identify, the biobank team leveraged the modern art of branding, wearing scrubs and hairnets in conspicuous bright pink and affixing kits to the door with pink tape. The biobank team also leveraged the art of simple human kindness, bringing snacks and goody-bags to the clinical staff and never failing to express gratitude.

As the relay continued, the runners delivered hundreds of samples to the lab each day for the processing team. Often putting in eleven-hour days, Esther Cheng, a master's degree candidate who redeployed to the biobank team, would float between running samples and doing lab work, wherever she was needed. Eventually, she led the RNA and DNA extractions and focused her work in a BSL-3 lab—including "pulling an all-nighter." "It was an eye-opening experience to see just how terrifying the virus was," said Ms. Cheng. "I'm very grateful that I was able to experience this emotional roller coaster—so much pain and illness, but I felt like I contributed to the healing process. I realized research is more than just the questions you're asking. It's about trying to make this world a better place, to give back to humanity."

As New York's frightening first wave began to recede, in mid-May, the biobank team had collected more than its initial ambitious goal of samples from 500 patients. The patient population was, mercifully, beginning to dwindle. At the same time, researchers were champing at the bit to have access to the data. Further, redeployed workers were starting to be called back to their previous positions. So Alex Charney and Miriam Merad decided to end the first phase of the biobank and transition to data generation. "It ended as quickly as it started," said Dr. Charney. "They were like these superheroes that just appeared in the night, came to the rescue, then went back to their day jobs."

The experience, he knew, would stay with them. With him, too.

"Permeating this whole project was—I don't know what the word is—almost like a religious experience," he said. "You just felt that what you were doing was so decent and good and right, that you were in the right place and there was no other place you should be other than where you were."

WITH SAMPLES PROCESSED and banked, next came the task of generating clinical and molecular data so researchers could access and study it—a task that the layperson might best appreciate in the sheer scope of a grid built by genomic and genetic scientist Noam Beckmann, which had about nine or ten iterations in its first several months. "The clinical table that everyone is using now has about, I want to say, 6,000 phenotypes by 25,000 individual time points," said Dr. Beckmann, whose work focuses on creating disease models by leveraging big data and advanced computational strategies. "It's a crazy table. It took an absurd amount of work to generate."

The idea was to see what is going on in the RNA, DNA, and other molecular components of any given patient at any given time, in any given situation, so researchers could investigate what was happening on a cellular level over time and over disease severity. The 6,000-by-25,000 clinical table enabled scientists to look at detailed molecular components in each cell (derived from the collected and processed blood samples) and compare them across subjects, across time periods, and across the all-important phenotype data, which refers to observable characteristics of each patient. *Did they live or die? Were they in the ICU? Were they intubated? How long were they in the hospital? What therapeutic interventions did they get and when?*

The early decisions on which phenotypes to include would define the biobank's ultimate usefulness, said Dr. Beckmann, which was why he put in fourteen-hour days seven days a week. "I will say that the quality of the scientific questions that you can ask are one hundred percent reliant on the quality of the phenotype data set that you have—so, time well spent, I believe," he said.

By way of example, he explained, "'ICU' was a really important phenotype for us in the design because it was important to try to understand the difference between people who ended up intubated in the ICU and the people who didn't. If we could understand it, maybe we could help solve it."

One researcher who put the data to work right away was Dr. Gnjatic. He sought to understand how quickly antibodies to COVID were generated, how durable they were, and what qualities they had. The data held some surprises. He had not expected, for instance, that most hospitalized patients would come in with a very robust antibody response. Why, then, he wondered, didn't those antibodies protect them from disease severe enough to require hospitalization?

So he pressed the data even further, following the quality and quantity of antibodies over time. The longitudinal nature of the study gave him a more kinetic and multidimensional understanding of antibody response. "We have samples from very early—upon admission—then every three days, and, eventually, long-term, as well," Dr. Gnjatic said. "We see the trajectories of the antibodies fall into different categories: those patients who start high and stay high, those patients who start low and become high, and those patients who start low and stay low. Their outcomes are quite different. It's a very interesting study, which we couldn't have done without this database."

Even as the pandemic continued to bear down on much of the world and Dr. Beckmann was in the midst of the data generation, he could envision researchers using the biobank to study diseases beyond COVID-19, as well. "We could use these data sets to really increase our understanding of how the genetic control of gene expression happens," he said, which ultimately defines how cells function and identity is expressed. As of mid-2021, the COVID-19 Biobank was available to all Mount Sinai researchers, and the team was investigating whether and how to make it accessible to the global scientific community.

"I don't know many data sets out there that have the longitudinal component in hundreds of individuals," Dr. Beckmann said. "In what [other] circumstance are you going to ask someone to come back and donate blood multiple days in a row? There's a richness to this data, biologically, that offers an incredible opportunity to learn things way beyond COVID."

PART 4

BUILDING THE FUTURE OF HEALTH CARE

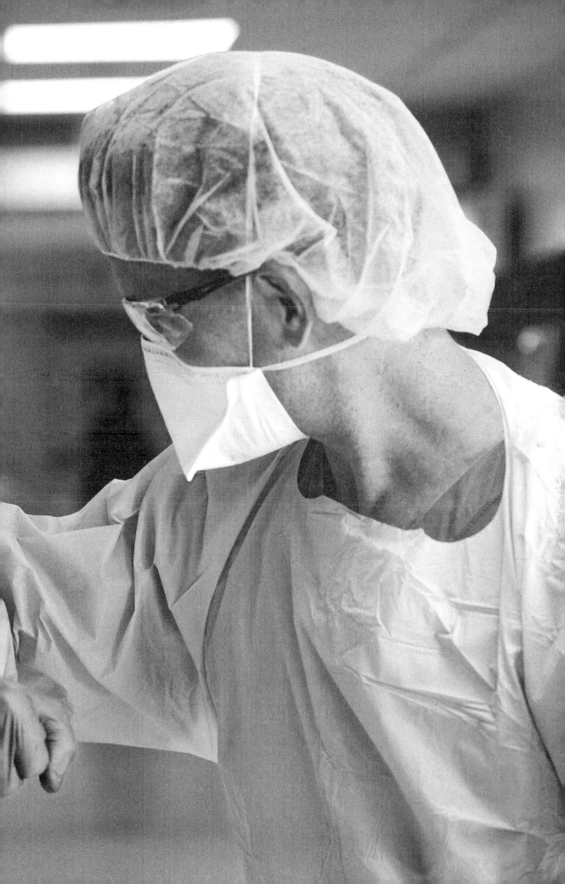

CHAPTER

13

WHAT THE PANDEMIC REVEALED

'We had an obligation to act'

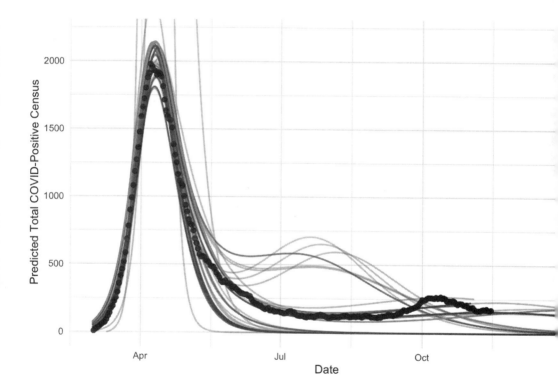

Above: Data scientists created a dynamic model to plan for the pandemic's peak patient census. Previous page: physician assistants Kristen Thoelen and Greg Montes give the typical pandemic greeting.

AS IT RIPPED THROUGH NEW YORK CITY and, soon enough, across the United States—which throughout 2020 suffered the most deaths in the world—COVID-19 laid bare the challenges, strengths, and weaknesses of the American health care system. From its vantage point in the center of the storm, and with a history of leading at medicine's progressive edge, Mount Sinai experienced the challenges earlier than most and responded in full force, building on foundations of strength to both respond immediately and begin to shape post-pandemic health care. Mount Sinai rapidly established several new programs to address needs that the pandemic had uncovered or, more often, elevated—needs that were known, were already being addressed to some degree. But the greatest exogenous shock in more than a century dramatically accelerated several trends already in motion.

"We acted very quickly to understand the disease better, to understand the consequences of the pandemic," said Dean Dennis Charney. "We put these findings into place almost immediately. We invested in understanding the effect of the disease on our frontline workers' mental health, in understanding why people of color were having worse outcomes, in developing a data center to inform diagnosis and treatment, and in systematically monitoring and analyzing the long-term impact of COVID. This was not only the right thing to do, we had an obligation to act—not only for us, but for the nation and for the world. We were the epicenter of the epicenter."

As it was caring for patients and conducting science, Mount Sinai was also aiming to shift the health care system, bending it toward racial equity and social justice, toward honoring health care workers as not just heroes but humans in need of help, and toward a true partnership with the patient, particularly in defining this novel disease, its symptoms and its acute and chronic impact. Mount Sinai was trying to ever shorten the bridge between medicine and science, leveraging big data and amplifying collaborations across all axes, including much-valued public-private partnerships. And it was moving flexibly and nimbly at a pace never before traveled in health care, and urging a new focus on cultivating resilience—of systems, spaces, stuff, and staff—to sustain itself and the people it serves in a decidedly uncertain future.

✢

HARNESSING BIG DATA:
INFORMING CARE IN REAL TIME

'The marriage of astute clinical observation with
analysis of harmonized data'

DATA SCIENTIST Bethany Percha saw just how much clinicians re-lied on her Mount Sinai COVID patient projections when she changed the Google link needed to access her daily forecast. Since late March, using a model of the SARS-CoV-2 infectious process in New York City, Dr. Percha had been creating forecasts of the number of COVID patients in Mount Sinai hospitals and ICUs currently and into the future, including estimating the date of the surge's projected peak and the number of patients expected to be hospitalized at that time.

The day of the new Google link, she received an email from a clinician who could not access the report and grew anxious without it. *Every morning when I get up, I look at this data,* he emailed. *It's my morning ritual.*

"This doctor was working with real COVID patients—why does he want to look at a graph?" Dr. Percha wondered at first. Then, the power of data, which was her livelihood, struck her anew. "Some-how, seeing the same data presented in a consistent way each day and seeing that things hadn't exploded overnight was helpful to him," she reflected. "That changed how I thought about my job. It was surprising to me as a science nerd just how comforting data are to people under conditions of uncertainty."

In January 2020, Dr. Percha had started a new role at Mount Sinai, establishing a data team within the department of medicine. When COVID hit, the head of the department, Barbara Murphy, was assidu-ously trying to prepare her units, to make sure there were enough beds and staff and resources for what was to come. But what was to come? The only outside models available at the time projected numbers that were, in Dr. Percha's words, "just apocalyptic": a peak in mid- to late April and numbers projected to be as high as 25,000 patients in Mount Sinai hospitals. How could clinical and operational leaders prepare for those kinds of numbers?

Dr. Murphy believed there had to be a model more representative of Mount Sinai's experience and more responsive to changes on the ground in New York City. So she asked Dr. Percha to create it. Building on the existing models, Dr. Percha created a dynamic model that incorporated the Health System's own data, including average length of hospital stay (approximately ten days, but ever shifting) and ICU stay (approximately twenty-one days), and took into account on-the-ground behavior in New York City, such as greater social distancing under the statewide lockdown, which reduced transmission.

Dr. Percha and many colleagues, including public health researchers Nick DeFelice and Allan Just, refined and revised the model, evolving its parameters to reflect what was happening on the ground. As they did, the COVID curve began to look a little less apocalyptic. Each day, the anticipated peak was revised downward from the earlier models' high of 25,000+ patients expected in late April, to the actual peak of just under 2,000 patients on April 10.

"What our model did for people was to provide a baseline for what our most likely scenario was going to be," Dr. Percha said, allowing that there was still a "great deal of uncertainty in all the parameters," given the pandemic's many unknowns. While she built the model for Dr. Murphy, its usefulness spread by word of mouth until Dr. Percha was sending it to some 50 people each day, including the clinician who read it as part of his morning ritual. "The alternative is you are literally staring at a graph that's going up and up and up, and you have no idea how far it's going to go up," said Dr. Percha. "That was terrifying."

DR. PERCHA'S WORK was part of Mount Sinai's massive data mobilization—which began pre-pandemic but accelerated profoundly during COVID—to inform clinical approaches, operational readiness, and scientific knowledge. There was desperate need for real-time data to help clinicians make pivotal decisions in the heat of battle with a novel virus about which little, at first, was known.

"The more we encountered COVID, the less we knew about it," said Girish Nadkarni, a nephrologist and data scientist who co-led, along with Alex Charney, a fast-proliferating group that would become the Mount Sinai Clinical Information Center (MSCIC) and would augment the role for data across the health system. "Early on, we realized that one thing we could do was bring all of the data together on a single platform, learn from it, and eventually inform the care of our patients."

Self-described "science nerds" like Dr. Percha, data gurus, and digital technology experts knew that Mount Sinai had a gold mine of data—particularly for the work at hand, COVID data. "Once you put data all together, once you have a good data set that's clean and well curated, there are a lot of questions you can ask," said Zahi Fayad, a pioneer in the fast-changing field of imaging and a leader in digital technology and artificial intelligence who helped MSCIC get off the ground. "That's how we started to ask all these questions, one after the other. So that's the story of the COVID kids," as he calls the largely young and always energetic group of researchers who made up the MSCIC.

Even before the mysterious virus surfaced in New York, Dr. Fayad and other radiologists had begun analyzing images and data from Chinese colleagues (as noted in Chapter 10) and describing early diagnosis insights and options. Then, in March, patients started streaming into New York hospitals, and Dr. Fayad asked, "Why don't we take that experience we had with China and see what we can do with the data that will be emerging from Mount Sinai? How can we, as scientists, leverage the data to do something useful—in real time, right now, right away?"

The first step in leveraging the data was to harmonize it. As with much of health care in the United States, Mount Sinai's data lived in several different systems. Radiology images were collected in one system, for example, and EKGs in another, explained Dr. Nadkarni. Scientists needed to locate what data was where, get permission to access it, then call in the data engineers to put it together in a framework that makes cohesive sense. And fast.

"I don't know if you realize how difficult it is," said Dr. Fayad. "It takes years to gather data from different sources and put them together in a single setup. And we did this in weeks."

Once the data streams lived together on a common platform, teams of researchers and clinicians could sleuth for patterns that began to tell a story—and to inform care. Data-driven discoveries included:

- Validating the widespread use of anticoagulants to treat COVID patients
- Illuminating just how big a problem acute kidney injury was, occurring in 46 percent of hospitalized COVID patients, 19 percent of whom required dialysis
- Revealing that more than one third of COVID patients suffered from myocardial injury and were at higher risk of death, or heart damage, that often accompanied COVID-19

In addition to interrogating data collected from patients across the health system, MSCIC scientists also analyzed data from health care workers—personalized data collected through wearables. Two MSCIC scientists, Dr. Fayad and Robert Hirten, explored how wearables might inform clinical care, and they made a headline-grabbing discovery. The pair created something called the Warrior Watch, an Apple watch that monitors users via vital sign measurement and an interactive app and symptom checker, to study the physical and mental health of hundreds of Mount Sinai health care workers who volunteered for the study. In one striking finding, the researchers noticed a significant change in the heart rate variability in participants who developed COVID-19. The changes were seen as many as seven days before people went on to test positive via a nasal swab.

"Developing a way to identify people who might be sick even before they know they are infected would really be a breakthrough in the management of COVID-19," said Dr. Hirten.

The Warrior Watch study also sought to analyze the psychological impact of the extended pandemic on health care workers. Enrolling

Mount Sinai health care workers across occupations—including a mix of those who were clinically trained and those who weren't—it monitored physiological and psychological signs of stress over time. The study found that emotional-support systems, quality of life, and resilience matter. Health care workers who reported higher measures of resilience and more emotional supports in their lives had not only lower levels of perceived stress but also a unique nervous system profile as measured by the Apple watch. This demonstrated that they were better protected against the psychological and physical effects of pandemic-related stress, according to the study published in September 2021, about a year and a half after Mount Sinai began receiving COVID-19 patients. These findings, said Drs. Fayad and Hirten, could help Mount Sinai—and other health care organizations—better understand who is most at risk of suffering from psychological effects of the pandemic and connect them to the mental health supports they need.

MOUNT SINAI'S "anticoagulation story," as many people referred to it, permeated through clinical care and data science from very early on in the pandemic. As described in Chapter 3, clinicians throughout the health system were noticing COVID patients clotting their dialysis tubes and presenting with surprising strokes and emboli. And, in record time, Mount Sinai created and disseminated a protocol for most COVID patients in Mount Sinai hospitals.

Then, of course, clinicians wanted to assess how well it was working. *Did it indeed prevent clotting?* Dr. Fuster and his colleagues wanted to know. *Who was benefiting? And when? Was it better to give treatment prophylactically, before clotting trouble surfaced, or as a therapeutic intervention?*

To observe outcomes in thousands of patients across Mount Sinai hospitals, Dr. Fuster turned to Dr. Nadkarni, whom colleagues call "the data science guru."

"He had the questions, and we had data and the scientific resources to address those question," said Dr. Nadkarni, who had worked closely with Dr. Fuster before and held the esteemed cardiologist as a mentor. Dr. Nadkarni and his team mined data to come up with answers on a remarkable timetable—in twenty-four hours.

"It was an all-hands-on-deck type of thing," said Dara Meyer, MSCIC's project leader who had the inside view on many collaborations. "This was urgent. This could really impact people. I don't think anybody slept during the entire first wave. We were burning the candle at both ends because we knew people's lives depended on it."

By analyzing electronic health record data on 4,389 COVID patients hospitalized between March 1 and April 30, investigators found that all regimens of anticoagulants were far better for patients than no blood thinners at all. Those who received anticoagulants—whether a full or lower dose—had about a 50 percent higher chance of survival and about a 30 percent lower chance of needing intubation.

"The importance of all these stories in my mind is the marriage of an astute clinical observation with analysis of harmonized data," said Dr. Nadkarni. "A big lesson learned is the value of our data, which shouldn't be locked in silos. We should be using all this data for our patients."

⁜

DRIVING HEALTH EQUITY: HOW TWIN CRISES BEGAN TO CHANGE THE EQUATION

'It's almost surreal that suddenly everybody's prepared to have this conversation'

Without health, you don't have the tools and resources to pursue any of your other liberties. It's the most basic human capacity. To have people sick because they're hungry and dying because they're not getting health care—that's not acceptable.

—LYNNE RICHARDSON, *co-director, Mount Sinai Institute for Health Equity Research*

———

WHEN A LONGTIME family friend arrived at the 2020 Zoom seder extremely short of breath, Carol Horowitz knew what she was looking at. "You need to call 911. Now," Dr. Horowitz told her friend, an older Black woman who had a number of underlying conditions in addition to the sudden respiratory symptoms that the doctor knew could mean COVID.

No, no, her friend said. She couldn't call 911, couldn't go to the hospital. "I don't have my wig on," she said.

"She *knows*," said Dr. Horowitz, a population health scientist and dean for gender equity in science.

This was not a question of vanity or triviality. Rather, said Dr. Horowitz, "She knows how people in the health care system can stigmatize overweight Black women on Medicaid."

When Dr. Horowitz and the rest of the family finally convinced the friend to call 911, she was taken to a local community hospital, not her usual Mount Sinai hospital. "She felt the doctors there were so discouraging that she saw no point in allowing them to intubate her. She feared that once on the ventilator she would never get off," Dr. Horowitz recounted. "And she died."

As a health equity researcher, Dr. Horowitz was well aware that a similar personal story played out over and over in countless families across New York City and across the country during the pandemic. Mount Sinai clinicians and researchers saw in the data—and in their hospitals—that COVID was devastating families and communities of color. According to the CDC, Black and Latinx Americans were nearly three times as likely as whites to be hospitalized due to COVID and twice as likely to die of the disease.

"Who gets COVID-19, who lives and who dies, maps very well, unfortunately, with other kinds of maps we have in New York City," said Dr. Horowitz, who would go on to become director of Mount Sinai's new Institute for Health Equity Research. "This includes areas of poverty, areas with a majority of low-income, Latinx, and Black people, areas of more pollution, areas of more linguistic isolation, areas that have had more redlining in the past and other structural inequities. If you look at any map of New York City and where people are marginalized, don't have equal opportunities, and have higher burdens of chronic diseases, these are the same areas where COVID-19 hit the hardest."

Founded on progressive values and with its foundational Manhattan hospital straddling one of the greatest disparities of ZIP codes in the country—both the wealthy Upper East Side and the largely immigrant and minority East Harlem neighborhoods—Mount Sinai had long been committed to quality care for all. But the pandemic would reveal how much more attention intractable inequities demanded. Department of Health numbers during New York City's first wave tell the story: in the 10029 ZIP code of East Harlem, there were 1,698 COVID-19 cases and 182 deaths; in the 10028 ZIP code, the Upper East Side, there were 603 cases and 34 deaths.

To health equity researchers, this disparity was far from a revelation. This was something they knew, had studied, had put numbers to for decades. "This was not new to COVID," said Lynne Richardson, an emergency physician and heath equity researcher who would become co-director of the institute. "This is true of hypertension and heart failure and kidney disease, diabetes, HIV, cancer. The list goes on and on with these disparities in outcomes."

But the starkness and cruelty of COVID collided with other factors during the pandemic to lay bare health care inequities and accelerate the pursuit of remedies. As COVID struck Black and Latinx communities especially hard, the nation faced a crisis of another sort, a racial reckoning spurred by George Floyd's murder—all this at a time when Americans were spending more time at home, under lockdown, and often glued to news. The layers of complexity, the sources of disparity were visible as the workforce bifurcated into people who could telework from home and those who had to report to jobs as essential workers, disproportionately people of color, putting them at greater risk of contracting COVID. And people in communities of color tend to live more to a household, in multigenerational or otherwise crowded apartments that put them at increased risk of spreading COVID.

It was, said Dr. Richardson, a tale of two cities.

In fact, Dr. Richardson lived this divide up close and personal, on the front lines of care. She split her time as an emergency department physician between the Mount Sinai Hospital in Manhattan and Elmhurst Hospital, one of the city's public hospitals, in Queens. As bad as things were in Mount Sinai hospitals, Elmhurst Hospital struggled even more mightily, inundated with patients in cramped spaces and strapped for resources at every turn.

IN MAY 2020, even before protests against systemic racism spread across the country, Mount Sinai—a medical school guided by values of social justice and equity and a hospital system that cares for a hugely diverse population—launched the Institute for Health Equity Research to change the equation. The new institute aimed to galvanize research and researchers across broad areas of study to focus through the lens of equity; and to build and educate a diverse work force, particularly in the areas of equity research. Richard Friedman, the Boards of Trustee co-chair, was a driving force behind both the philanthropy that made the institute possible and the luminaries recruited to its outside task force, including Magic Johnson of basketball and business fame; Ruth Simmons, former president of Brown University; and financiers, politicians, and media executives—people who, as Mr. Friedman said, "could really shout the message out to the world."

Such an institute, said Dr. Richardson, accelerates health equity research in a way that can, realistically, translate to impact. "These transdisciplinary research institutes are the Sinai model for how you investigate the most important questions in science, the most important areas of discovery," said Dr. Richardson. "To have this model now focused on health equity science was really an amazing development. To suddenly have the work we were doing elevated to the level of a research institute with a corresponding level of support and investment from the institution was quite breathtaking. It's almost surreal that suddenly everybody's prepared to have this conversation, to invest in trying to understand problems that we've had for so long."

She marveled at how much the national conversation had already advanced. In the summer of 2021, she and Dr. Horowitz were busy putting together a grant for a funding opportunity put out by the National Institutes of Health on understanding the impact of structural racism. "Two years ago," said Dr. Richardson, "I would have bet you any amount of money that the NIH would never issue a document that had 'structural racism' in the title."

The institute will help Mount Sinai recruit researchers at all levels and from all backgrounds—and collaborate with a wide range of scientists across Mount Sinai—to deepen the study of health equity and find solutions to deep-seated challenges. "Health disparities are very complex," Dr. Richardson said. "They're biological, they're genetic, they're environmental, they involve social determinants, they involve health care. We need scientists from every discipline to help us think about and understand how health disparities work and how we eliminate them to achieve health equity. That's how we're going to solve this—bringing everybody to the table to think about these complex problems, as challenging in their own way as molecular discoveries."

Another priority is to learn directly from and partner with communities. In one of its first such partnerships, the institute launched a survey of what it hopes will be some 10,000 New Yorkers to learn more about their COVID experiences and link them to community resources. The survey asked about not only direct health impacts of the virus but also indirect health consequences.

After all, said Dr. Richardson, the fallout from the pandemic was broad and deep. People went without needed medical care and medication for diabetes, hypertension, congestive heart failure, and other chronic conditions. Inactivity exacerbated obesity. Mental health suffered. People experienced joblessness and food and housing insecurity. "Every single condition that we've ever studied is now worse because of COVID," Dr. Richardson said, adding that Mount Sinai and community-based partners were collaborating on ways to bring culturally appropriate mental health care to hard-hit communities of color.

"It's simply unacceptable to have people dying at disparate rates from COVID or high blood pressure or anything," said Dr. Richardson. "We certainly have to learn from our past, but it is about the path forward and there's so much work to be done. I am hopeful in a way that I haven't been in a long time, that maybe we will make some real progress in this country."

THE MOUNT SINAI HOSPITAL, CIRCA 2016—In her role with Mount Sinai's Office of Diversity and Inclusion (ODI), Pamela Abner was giving a workshop on unconscious bias to a group of administrators, largely people of color, she recalled, many of whom worked in patient registration. She had been talking about how people of color suffer disproportionately lousy outcomes in the U.S. health care system, and she asked the administrators how they inquire about and record patient information on race and ethnicity. "They looked at me as if I'd flown in from Mars," said Ms. Abner, who would go on to become vice president and chief diversity operations officer. They said they were told not to worry about capturing the data, to just mark down *unknown*.

"That was absolutely the opposite of what the institution should have been doing," said Ms. Abner, who since then has made it a mission to educate employees throughout Mount Sinai's health system on the importance of capturing data as a necessary step in making change. She noticed—to her horror—that some forms still listed as categories of race and ethnicity "Negro" and "Chicano."

"I realized nobody was really paying attention to this," she said. From then on, *she* was.

Fast-forward to 2020, when the pandemic struck people of color with a disproportionate brutality. There was a new urgency to revamp those data fields and educate employees and patients on why data collection was important and how it could affect outcomes, inform research, and ultimately reduce health disparities. In partnership with the new institute and data scientists, Ms. Abner convened a team that included Lyndia Hayden, ODI's director of disparities and analytics; Doran Ricks, a vice president for the health system who leads enterprise reporting; and Damon Myers from information technology.

Together, they created new dashboards. Gone was the *unknown* category (although patients had a *prefer not to respond* option). And nuance mattered. If someone identified as Black or African American, could they further identify a country of origin? Did people of Haitian descent, for instance, have certain outcomes or suffer certain disparities? "That information was very important to our clinicians and researchers who were studying communities where the disease was more prevalent," explained Ms. Abner. "Encouraging people to provide that specificity would help us as an academic research organization, so that we would be able to say what's going on in our communities."

"You don't know unless you know, right?" said Dr. Horowitz. By gathering information on race and ethnicity, researchers and clinicians can begin to ask questions, make connections, and enact solutions. "Do the data show a difference in processes, quality, or outcomes of care?" she asked. "If so, why? And let's fix it."

The slicing and dicing will go beyond race and ethnicity. Mount Sinai has begun geocoding patients, which means linking addresses to outcomes, looking at people in the context of their lived experiences. "So we're not only going to ask whether Black people or Latinx people or Asian people are more vulnerable or suffering negative outcomes," said Dr. Horowitz. "We're also going to be looking based on whether people are living in a neighborhood with higher crime, higher pollution, more linguistic isolation, less walkability. What are the factors in your neighborhood that might be making you sicker? Only ten or twenty percent of health has anything to do with health care. If we really want people to be healthy, what are we doing in their communities?"

✢

RESILIENCE AT WORK
'The best of times, the worst of times'

Resilience is typically thought of as an individual-level trait and refers to one's ability to do just what it sounds like—to bend but not break, to be pushed but bounce back. And yet we all have our limits—everybody can be bent to a breaking point. At the same time, everybody is resilient to a degree. My work focuses on creating a system that enables someone to use their resilience when needed, flourish in their environment, and derive meaning from their work. We're also trying to cultivate a workplace that

makes people feel supported and—particularly in times of crisis—a place where people know the institution has their back.
—JONATHAN RIPP, *chief wellness officer*

———

"I THINK ABOUT emotions as being something that has a beginning, middle, and end," said Gabrielle Finley, a social worker who ran one of the eleven-week workshops at the Mount Sinai Center for Stress, Resilience, and Personal Growth.

"They start out slowly, and then they have this crest, and if you let them pass and roll out, you'll get through the emotion," Ms. Finley told the Road to Resilience podcast. "Emotions don't last forever. But we tend to intervene. We don't let them run their full course. And when we do that, they just keep crashing on us and keep crashing on us. So there's no way to get past the emotion unless you swim through it."

Shauna Linn, a physician assistant who was redeployed to COVID-19 units and who participated in the workshops, said, "You're not going to solve your whole life issue in an hour once a week, but it gives you strategies, tools. It provides a safe space for open communication. It invites you to be with people who you might not cross paths with otherwise but who have a similar motivation and desire to hash out these questions."

Jonathan DePierro, the center's clinical director who had served as supervising psychologist at the Icahn School of Medicine at Mount Sinai World Trade Center Mental Health Program, said about the evidence-based workshops, "The word *resilience* is very important right now because so many staff faced adversity in the peak of the pandemic. It really challenges how people cope, how people view themselves, the world, other people, how safe they feel. We really need to build on our strengths and capitalize on our resilience to help us adapt to this new normal."

The center offered confidential screening for mental health risk, as well as treatment at no cost to Mount Sinai employees, said Deborah Marin, a psychiatrist who co-directs the center. Programming also included training peer leaders within the health system and in the community and a buddy system for nurses to check in on one another's well-being. In collaboration with the Hasso Plattner Digital Health Institute at Mount Sinai, the center created an app to track resilience and psychosocial risks, provide daily interventions, and connect users to care if further interventions are needed. And Mount Sinai scientists were conducting ongoing research into the molecular makeup and bio-determinants of stress, risk, and resilience, seeking to improve diagnosis and treatment. Recent research included a study by neuroscientist Scott Russo on stress, coping strategies, and resilience in animal models; a study by James Murrough, associate professor of neuroscience and psychiatry who directs the Depression and Anxiety Center for Discovery and Treatment, on new neuroscientific targets for treating stress disorders; and the Warrior Watch study by Drs. Fayad and Hirten.

Dean Charney, a Bruce Springsteen fan, took the center's motto from a Springsteen song, *We take care of our own.* "We must help them recover to ensure the future of our health care system," Dean Charney said.

IN HIS STUDIES on resilience, Dean Charney has seen how fear can guide—rather than paralyze—people in uncommonly dangerous situations. He has spoken with POWs from the Vietnam War, Navy Seals, members of the Delta Force, and others whose resilience was seriously tested. Were they fearless, as their job might suggest? he wondered. "No, no," they said, telling him, "Of course we feel fear. We let fear guide us, and we learn how to handle the fear. Our training kicks in, and we learn from fear."

Facing fear is one of ten resilience factors Dean Charney and Steven Southwick, emeritus professor at Yale School of Medicine, have outlined in their research—research that informs the new center's evidence-based workshops and programs. Dean Charney saw this factor playing out as Mount Sinai workers battled the deadly virus. "They let the fear guide the way they handled the patient," Dean Charney said in an interview in the fall of 2020. "They were careful, they didn't get infected. Even though they were afraid, their training kicked in."

Dean Charney described other resilience factors that he saw at work on the floors of the hospitals, in support roles behind the scenes, and in busy labs, including:

- Working together in common purpose, guided by a moral compass: "They felt tremendous pride that they had done the right thing at great personal risk," Dean Charney said. "For the rest of their lives, the pride and the competence they felt will help in the inevitable challenges they'll face."
- Trusting training and experience: "Even when they were redeployed to another area, they knew they had the training, competence, and experience to do the work."
- Summoning optimism: "Not a Pollyanna optimism, but realistic optimism. '*Okay, I was trained for this, I can do this.*'"
- Receiving physical and emotional support: "It was very important that we provided not only the support materials—including personal protective equipment—but we also provided support emotionally."
- Finding resilient role models: "Support includes having role models to guide you through this journey."

"It was the best of times and the worst of times," Dean Charney said, reflecting on how health care workers rose to the challenge of a lifetime.

That takeaway is echoed by health care workers throughout these pages. One such worker, Dayna McCarthy, spoke on her thirty-eighth birthday about how she, as a young doctor, was becoming disillusioned by what medicine had become but how her passion was reignited during the pandemic—despite working around the clock, getting COVID herself, and struggling still with post-acute COVID. The intense, immediate, and highly collaborative work reminded her why she went into medicine in the first place—to care directly and urgently for patients, rather than getting mired in the ever-increasing bureaucracy and paperwork of health care. "Sometimes it feels like there's so much between me and the patient care—like it's ten percent about caring for the patient and ninety percent about all the stuff in between," she said. "Now, it was so pared down. It was all about the patient. As terrible as it was, I felt grateful for the experience. And it's why I went into medicine."

Dr. Richardson, the health equity researcher who treated patients in the emergency departments at Mount Sinai and Elmhurst hospitals, also suffered through COVID-19 at home for a couple weeks and got right back to work: "There was simply no choice but to keep going because every day there were, again, hundreds of sick patients waiting for you. It was a very, very difficult time."

And, at the same time, she said, "I've really never been more proud to be an emergency physician. My colleagues rallied—all of us, the attending physicians, resident physicians, nurses, nursing assistants, techs, we all came to work every day, putting our own health at risk, and the health of our families at risk. It was tremendous that everybody was just focused on saving as many lives as we could."

JONATHAN RIPP has been Mount Sinai's chief wellness officer since 2018, responsible for the medical school's increased focus on the well-being of students, residents and fellows, and faculty physicians and scientists—people who, even outside a pandemic, experience a significant amount of stress. The emotional and psychological distress of the health care workforce—or, more accurately, *reducing* that distress—was in his wheelhouse. Early in the pandemic, Dr. Ripp and colleagues at Stanford chronicled the sources of anxiety among health care workers in a paper published online in the *Journal of the American Medical Association* on April 7, 2020. Dr. Ripp and the team stratified the needs into five categorical requests that health care workers had for their institutions: *hear me, protect me, prepare me, support me, care for me.* Those needs became something of a refrain, Dr. Ripp found; he heard them invoked by other health care organizations putting together their own employee mental health supports.

At first, early in the pandemic, Dr. Ripp noted, health care workers' main concerns were about meeting their basic daily needs. *Will there be enough personal protective equipment to keep me safe? Will I put my loved ones at risk? Who will watch my children? How will I get to work?* Even, *Where will my next meal come from?* "We partnered across the system with human resources, psychiatry, social work, and spiritual care to very rapidly develop both information and resources to address those basic daily needs," Dr. Ripp said. Mount Sinai connected employees to temporary housing, free parking, access to child care, meals—so many meals—and other basic needs, as well as mobilized on many fronts to procure and distribute PPE.

The true extent of psychological fallout often happens after trauma, in this case after the waves of the most intense pandemic care. "In the midst of crisis, people just hunker down and get the job done," said Dr. Ripp. "But once things calm down and you can take a breath, that's when you begin to reflect on what you've been through. It can be a very delicate time."

A recent Mount Sinai study of more than 4,000 World Trade Center responders bore this out. Twelve-plus years after the 2001 trauma, 26.8 percent of police and 46 percent of nontraditional responders still reported suffering from some degree of WTC-related PTSD.

Crisis creates opportunity, as many stories in these pages demonstrate, and one of Dr. Ripp's areas of focus is what's called "post-traumatic growth." That includes highlighting the profound meaning of the work done against long odds during the greatest health care challenge in a century. "By drawing attention to the impact our workforce had during the crisis, to the difference they made, we believe we can shift them away from post-traumatic stress and toward post-traumatic growth," said Dr. Ripp. "That would mean they could look back on this experience as one of the most meaningful things they've done in their career, a time when they were most needed and were able to bring their skills to bear on something so challenging."

DAVID PUTRINO, who studies rehabilitation and resilience among high-performance athletes and elite military operators, believes that an important takeaway from the pandemic for all organizations—especially health care organizations—is their role in nurturing resilience. Resilience is not only an individual pursuit, he emphasized, but a communal effort.

"The newest literature around resilience tells us that it's a social resource," said Dr. Putrino, who created Mount Sinai's recharge rooms. "If you want a resilient workplace, you need to make a humane workplace. You need to signal with everything that you have that you're looking after your people. Our responsibility to all of the workers who put everything on the line during the pandemic is to be that organization for them—to signal that we have their back, that we're going to provide every single service we can to keep them feeling healthy and help them move past the trauma that they've experienced. That's how you build a resilient workforce."

For students who were about to enter a career plagued by high levels of burnout and who experienced tremendous upheaval during the pandemic, the Icahn School of Medicine began shifting the conversation from "well-being" to talk of individual and communal resilience, acknowledging that it is okay to *not* feel well in overwhelming circumstances. Alicia Hurtado, associate dean for medical student wellness and student affairs, said that the school's support system focused on normalizing the experience of feeling distinctly *unwell*, of honoring grief and sadness, in times of so much pain and loss. "We emphasized that it is important to experience such emotions in order to process loss," Dr. Hurtado wrote in a paper prepared for the Josiah Macy Jr. Foundation Conference on COVID-19 and the Impact on Medical and Nursing Education held in July 2021. "Our school's medical education community needed to acknowledge the feeling in the air: of hospital wards not always being a place of triumph and success; of medical school and medical practice sometimes feeling futile; of how our shared experiences with sadness, grief, and exhaustion made us stronger by virtue of being shared."

SHAPING POST-ACUTE COVID CARE

'I don't know, but I'm here to support you'

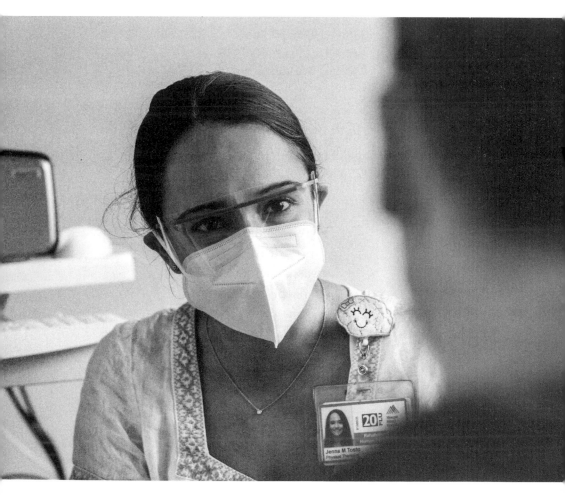

To care for people with devastating lingering symptoms, Mount Sinai built the first-of-its-kind interdisciplinary Center for Post-COVID Care.

MAY 17, 2020—A loud thumping sound woke Nitza Rochez in the middle of the night. She was dizzy, had a terrible headache, and slowly realized that the loud thumping was her heart. She went to the emergency room, something she as a healthy young woman was not used to doing. She registered extremely high blood pressure (as opposed to her normally low BP) but no other measurable threats, and was told she was fine. It was anxiety. Go home, sleep it off.

She went to the ER another ten or so times, including later that same day, and was told ten or so times that she was fine. That was despite her mounting symptoms, which also included pulsing in her spine, tremors in her hands, and violently shaking vision. Her legs felt heavy, encased in cement. "I honestly thought that I was dying," said Ms. Rochez, who had been a marathon runner and worked in corporate branding, neither of which she has been able to do since getting sick. "There's no way to feel so just completely unwell every single hour of every day and not be dying."

Ms. Rochez had had COVID in March—a bad bout, but she was not hospitalized and seemed to recover after a few weeks. But she didn't connect these new, strange symptoms to the novel virus. Neither did the emergency room doctors (at a New York City hospital that was not a Mount Sinai hospital). COVID had been present in the United States for only a couple months (at least visibly; likely, it had been circulating longer). The focus was, understandably, on the ravages of acute COVID. The world was so deeply *mid*; few people were talking yet about *post*.

At her last emergency room visit, in June, she saw her life coming to an end. Not because she was so tired and weak and suffered physical and visual tremors. But because of what the doctor said in the face of those symptoms.

"You're fine," he told her. Again. "It's all in your head."

"He's telling me I'm fine as the image of him is literally shaking wildly," Ms. Rochez recalled. She felt she must be going crazy, so overwhelmed was she by ruinous symptoms that no one else seemed to see.

"So I went back home," she said, thinking, "I'm just going to die."

MEANWHILE, rehab scientist David Putrino and neuroscientist Christopher Kellner had reconfigured an electronic tool they'd developed to monitor stroke patients at home to now monitor and triage COVID patients at home. These were people who were not sick enough to be hospitalized—at least, not yet—but were still pretty sick with COVID symptoms (whether or not they'd had a positive PCR test, as tests were then hard to come by). The novel virus had confounded clinicians and scientists in so many ways, and the app allowed health care workers to monitor people's vital signs and symptoms remotely, to see when someone took a turn for the worse and required hospitalization. This was proving to be an effective way to manage care in a time when patients were proliferating, beds were limited, and people wanted to avoid going to hospitals if they could.

But amid the anticipated outcomes, monitoring patients and getting them to the hospital when needed, Drs. Putrino and Kellner also found something they hadn't anticipated—something that would help write the pandemic's next chapter and ultimately give hope to people like Nitza Rochez.

"There was about 10 percent of the cohort we monitored, 30 or 40 people, who just weren't getting better," Dr. Putrino said, adding that he and his colleagues were already starting to doubt the CDC's relative clarity that COVID symptoms should recede after about two weeks. "This group of patients couldn't quite shake it, and they were developing new symptoms: *I'm really tired. I can't leave the house. My heart is racing.*"

Even as clinicians and scientists were working quickly to save acutely ill patients from dying, physicians started to notice what Drs. Putrino and Kellner had: people who had recovered from the acute phase of the illness were still suffering from lingering, debilitating symptoms. Fatigue, brain fog, extreme weakness, mental health issues, kidney problems, and the list goes on. Given the heterogeneity of the illness, the still largely black box of its pathophysiology, and the fact that there was no study yet of the aftermath of an illness brand new to humankind, there were vastly more questions than answers. But it was becoming increasingly clear that for a meaningful number of people, COVID-19 would go on to become a chronic, disabling illness.

In a retrospective observational study, Drs. Kellner, Putrino, and several colleagues analyzed 84 patients with what they were calling post-acute COVID syndrome (PACS), and found symptoms lasted from 54 to 255 days. Almost all of the patents, 92 percent, suffered from fatigue, and most reported loss of concentration or memory, weakness, headache, dizziness, and reduced quality of life.

"Long-lasting symptoms not yet defined by any current diagnostic paradigm can be extremely daunting for patients and give rise to a sense of isolation," the authors noted in their paper, put up on a preprint server in November 2020. "As such, clinicians are urged to acknowledge the presence of the persistent symptoms that can impact the health and well-being of patients with PACS."

By virtue of volume and vigilance, Mount Sinai became the earliest health care system to identify and build a program to address the many and varied persistent symptoms associated with long-term COVID, working on both clinical care and research. The Center for Post-COVID Care launched in May 2020 to provide personalized, multispecialty care to affected patients, while also gathering clinical data on a disease about which clinicians and researchers know so little.

The head of the center, endocrinologist Zijian Chen, said doctors estimated that 30 percent of people who'd had COVID would go on to suffer from a variety of chronic conditions, including increased risk of thromboembolic disease, cardiovascular complications, liver and kidney problems, and systemic inflammatory dysfunction. In addition, severe acute COVID could result in mental health issues such as post-traumatic stress disorder, anxiety, and depression.

Building on a model that Mount Sinai created to provide medical and psychological care to World Trade Center responders, care begins with an extensive evaluation at the Center for Post-COVID Care, and then draws in many specialties. "After the initial intake, we have the flexibility to include different specialties, depending on what the patient needs," Dr. Chen said. "We have cardiology and pulmonary working with us, and neurology. Behavioral health services were needed—we expected a lot of depression and anxiety. We talked to rehab because we felt that the patients have deconditioning from their illness. We brought in an ENT [ear, nose, and throat] because so many people complained they couldn't smell or taste."

Mount Sinai leaders fashioned the seven-floor medical pavilion at 10 Union Square East into the country's first center for post-COVID care. The downtown location could be easily reached by almost every New York City subway line. The building—which had opened as a newly designed set of practices in March 2020 before closing weeks later and reopening as the post-COVID care center—houses many interconnected spaces, ideal for delivering interconnected care. "It's all located in one place, so the patient doesn't have to go to different places in order to find the care they need," said Dr. Chen. This was vital to patients who needed to meet with a primary care doctor, see a variety of specialists, and receive physical therapy, who might be coming from out of town, who had difficulty getting around, and who might need assistance attending their appointments.

Clinicians and researchers were eager to join the effort. "We needed to learn it, and the only way we can do that is to see a lot of patients," Dr. Chen said of the little-understood illness that was fast becoming the next big story in COVID care and science. "This is one of the largest multidepartmental collaborations within the system. There are a lot of people coming together to help one specific group of patients. This shows how far we can take something if we put our minds and our efforts together."

Dayna McCarthy, who treated post-acute COVID patients and had also led acute-COVID teams (read more in Chapter 2), described it as a new way of working, embracing the unknown in close collaboration across disciplines and, effectively, as committed apprentices to the illness. "I don't think there is going to be a eureka moment, a single fix," she said. "This is so multifactorial. We're going to glean so much information about the different systems of the body because so much is unknown. That's what COVID has taught us—there's so much we don't know. Especially about the immune system. We thought HIV taught us so much. This is the next step in the teaching."

A COUPLE OF DAYS after Nitza Rochez headed home from the ER for the last time, convinced that this unexplained illness was going to kill her, her sister called. She had just seen on the news that Mount Sinai had opened a post-COVID care center. "Nitza," her sister said, "this has to be post-COVID."

The earliest appointment at the busy center was August, and Nitza awaited the visit with equal parts anticipation and trepidation. "Even though it was a post-COVID care center," she said in an interview nearly a year later, "I was afraid I was going to get the same reaction: *I'm healthy, I'm young, I'm fit, this is all in my head.* I just figured I was in this on my own."

Her fear, it turned out, could not have been further from the truth. From the instant she walked with her cane through the doors of the Mount Sinai Center for Post-COVID Care, "I had the most amazing experience," Ms. Rochez recalled. "I would not be surprised if I cried in the appointment." Not only did the doctor seem to understand and validate every symptom, said Ms. Rochez, "she practically finished my sentences for me."

The doctor, Joan Bosco, asked her if she had any strange sensations when she woke up in the morning. "I had not shared this with any doctors because I thought they'd really think I was crazy," Ms. Rochez said. "When I would get up from bed or just stand up throughout the day, I would feel this sensation of numbness and heaviness start from my head all the way down to my toes."

Far from thinking her patient was crazy, the doctor said, "Yes, some patients are mentioning that, something that feels like a waterfall."

"That was the perfect description!" Ms. Rochez said. "I almost started crying because at that moment I knew: *Oh, my God, this is really real, it's not in my head, and I'm not alone.*"

After listening to Ms. Rochez's symptoms and taking every one of them seriously, Dr. Bosco and a team that included a physiatrist and neurologist built a treatment plan. Steroids, blood pressure medication (prescribed earlier), an anti-inflammatory diet to help with headaches, compression socks and pants to help with neuropathy, physical therapy, breathing techniques.

"The most important thing we do when they come in is allow them to be heard," said Dr. McCarthy. "That wasn't something they were getting before coming here. People were cutting them off, not wanting to hear what they had to say."

To even begin to understand and treat this puzzling illness, doctors had to listen fully to patients, and they had to do something often anathema to medicine: they had to say, *I don't know.*

"As doctors, as scientists, as human beings, we are humbled by what we don't know," Dr. McCarthy said. "To see patients suffering like this and not be able to help, it's humbling, it brings you to your knees. But to be able to say to a patient sitting there in front of you, 'I don't know, but I'm here to support you and help you. As soon as we know things, we're going to let you know'—that reaches out and touches them. They say to us, 'That's what I need in this moment. I just need somebody to say that to me, because I don't want to be in this on my own.'"

Dr. McCarthy brought another dimension to her understanding. She was also a patient.

Somewhere in caring for acute COVID patients at the Mount Sinai Hospital, she had come down with COVID herself—"a run-of-the-mill young-person COVID," she called it, which sidelined her with a sore throat, bad headaches, and loss of smell and taste. But, as is par for the post-acute COVID course, her recovery was soon followed by a bone-weary fatigue (*exertional malaise* is the technical term) that made her feel like she'd been hit by a truck. At first she chalked it up to the fact that she had been sick and was working too hard. "I was working my butt off, until like four in the morning," she said. Even when she had been quarantining with suspected COVID, she was remotely monitoring patients and managing admissions and discharges.

But her symptoms persisted. And worsened. Exhaustion, splitting headaches, brain fog, "couldn't exercise for the life of me," said the avid runner. "I knew what these patients were going through because I knew something was not right with me also. I had so much empathy."

Into the summer of 2021, she was still struggling to find the right treatment plan, combining medication with adjunctive therapies including acupuncture and craniosacral therapy, and taking one day at a time.

EVEN IF DOCTORS have few answers, the power of a diagnosis cannot be overestimated.

"I have POTS and dysautonomia," Caitlin Barber said matter-of-factly, knowledgeable about every aspect of postural orthostatic tachycardia syndrome (POTS) and the more generalized nervous system disorder, dysautonomia. "What that means is COVID damaged a part of my nervous system, my autonomic nervous system. Your autonomic nervous system does everything automatic in your body—your heart rate, blood pressure, temperature, digestion, sweat, everything that you don't have to think about. Even to the point that my eyes don't dilate and constrict appropriately."

The diagnosis, which brought her both fear and hope, was extremely hard won and represented a giant step forward. For months, all she knew was that she could barely move, and no one could tell her what was wrong. She, too, was a former marathon runner, and now she was so weak that she could not get out of bed, change clothes, or shower without considerable help. She couldn't return to her work as a registered dietician in a nursing home and barely left her small Hudson Valley apartment. When she did, she used a wheelchair.

Like Ms. Rochez's, Ms. Barber's health care odyssey kept meeting dead ends. No one linked it to the mild COVID she'd had in April 2020. "Nobody had an answer for me," she said. "Everybody was telling me I should be better by now because COVID is a two-week virus. *Why are you still sick? Are you sure this isn't anxiety?*"

Everybody, that is, except the Facebook COVID support group Survivor Corps, which has almost 170,000 members and which Ms. Barber finally found through dogged internet research into her symptoms. There, she learned about Mount Sinai's Center for Post-COVID Care. She got the next appointment she could, a month away, and in that month, her symptoms, including her heart rate, revved up so much that one night she Googled *What does a heart attack feel like?* "I'm twenty-seven years old, and I'm having a freaking heart attack?" she said, describing her state of disbelief.

Her husband called 911, and she was rushed to the emergency room with convulsions and seizures, which clinicians posited was a drug overdose. No one, she said, would entertain a conversation about post-COVID, but she held fast to her self-diagnosis—which would soon become a validated diagnosis. "I told them, 'I'm going to Mount Sinai this week. They have a post-COVID care center there. This is post-COVID.' They thought I was absolutely nuts. Sent me home. A couple days later, we go to Mount Sinai, and our world changed."

There, Dr. Bosco and a cardiologist spent hours with Ms. Barber and her husband. Every symptom she mentioned—which would ultimately number more than one hundred; she kept a list—was met with recognition and understanding. Common post-COVID issues, she was told. "Everybody up here in the Hudson Valley thought I was crazy, and when I went down there, they understood it," she said. "They knew what was happening with my body. They were so knowledgeable about post-COVID. And they answered our questions."

All except one—the biggest one of all. "They were very honest about the questions they could not answer," she said. *"Will I ever get better?"*

Doctors prescribed a high-salt high-fluid diet, compression socks, breath work, and physical therapy to restart her autonomic nervous system. She has gotten stronger and has gone back to work, though her activity is still limited.

As for Ms. Rochez, the constant headaches slowly lifted, and she began to move again. Initially, she was frustrated by how incremental the improvements were. "I ran for four and a half hours straight in the Brooklyn Marathon," she said, invoking her pre-pandemic life. "And now, just lifting my leg and putting it down in physical therapy drained me for the rest of the day. I would literally have to sleep it off as if I just ran."

But some ten months after her first visit, she was walking without a cane and could clock a quarter mile twice a day. Not the Brooklyn Marathon, but progress. "I have to learn to compare myself to where

I was a month ago, and a month before that," she said, speaking by Zoom from a holistic village retreat in Honduras, where she was spending some time to heal. The waking "waterfall sensation" was no longer there every time she stood, although she still had flareups, including tremors, weakness, and what she called "coughing madness." She set herself a goal: to be running by summer. It felt like a victory to even let herself begin saying that—"I will be running again."

"Honestly," said Ms. Rochez, "the fact that the doctors (A) listened, (B) came up with a plan, and (C) adjusted as needed—that made all the difference."

In June of 2021, the Centers for Disease Control and Prevention included in its comprehensive new standards of care for post-COVID one of the cardinal rules pioneered at Mount Sinai. "It is important for healthcare professionals to listen to and validate patients' experiences," said the CDC guidelines, "recognizing that diagnostic testing results may be within normal ranges even for patients whose symptoms and conditions negatively impact their quality of life, functioning ... and ability to return to school or work."

15

MOVING
FORWARD

'Putting it all to work for patients'

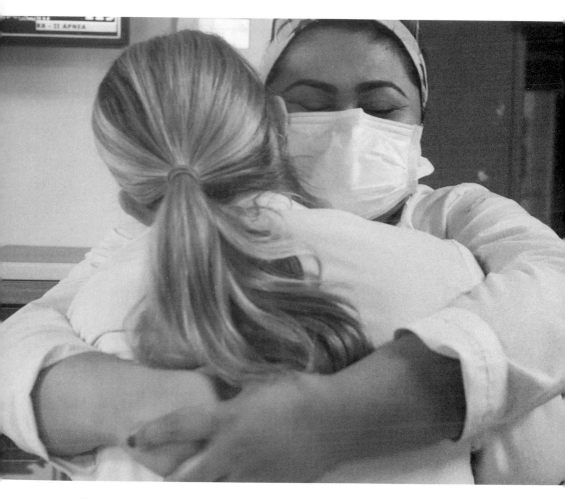

The pandemic demanded an unprecedented level of collaboration and compassion, an all-hands-on-deck urgency to treat, discover, and remain safe.

THE COVID-19 PANDEMIC DEALT—and, as of this writing, is still dealing—modern health care systems and health care workers the greatest test they've ever faced. There has been an unfathomable amount of loss and grief. But amid so much pain and personal sacrifice, Mount Sinai's health care workers banded together to save the lives of nearly 4,700 patients in the month of April 2020 alone, and would go on to treat and discharge a total of 7,700 in New York City's three-month first wave. That number grew to more than 11,700 by the end of January 2021.

Mount Sinai went beyond simply trying not to be overwhelmed: It innovated in the breech. "Mount Sinai was applying science and showing improved outcomes with therapeutic innovations in a way that demonstrated we are one of the best institutions in the world, especially with regard to COVID-19 care," said David Reich. "The Icahn School of Medicine, with its top scientists, was completely in lockstep with the largest health system in New York City. We were able to do things together that we never would have been able to do separately."

Building on existing partnerships and developing new ones, the people of Mount Sinai drew on training and well-honed expertise to learn, discover, and deliver care. They summoned deep wells of courage and compassion, flexibility and daring. They faced mounting numbers without fear or favor. They thought big and acted boldly, summoning everything they had—and considerable things that were not even in existence until they dreamed them up—to make inroads against a disease that could sometimes feel like it had them surrounded.

Jeremy Boal likened the kinetic discoveries to productivity in wartime. "The challenge is so overwhelming that you're just throwing everything at it that has an inkling of a chance to work. That's why there are so many innovations in wartime," said Dr. Boal. "We're learning, we're developing, we're putting it all to work for patients."

Days and nights have been long and trying. Supplies and space were in short supply, especially during the first wave, and expanding them demanded creativity and collaboration. The emotional and physical toll on patients, families, and health care workers continues to unspool. But there has been and continues to be discovery, too, and progress, new ways of working—developed in real time, often against audaciously long odds, to navigate a pandemic that seemed to write its own rules.

Throughout this book, Mount Sinai's health care workers detailed opportunities created, or amplified, in the pandemic that can inform and guide the health care system into the future. Those opportunities, largely overlapping and interwoven, include collaboration on a whole new order of magnitude; an accelerated pace of advancing medicine and science; innovation in care delivery models; and a renewed focus on preparedness and resilience, including the emotional well-being of health care workers.

✣

UNPRECEDENTED COLLABORATION

'It's a story of ... strategizing together'

THE FIGHT AGAINST coronavirus was at once a solitary battle and a solidary one. Day to day, minute by minute, it was deeply isolating. Patients were separated from loved ones in their most trying times. Frontline workers and biomedical researchers were ensconced in an armor of PPE. The whole world was taking its measure by six feet of distance. And yet, a health care crisis of pandemic proportion could not be fought alone, not by a single person, not by a single discipline, and not by a single hospital or health system, region or country.

Before the pandemic, Mount Sinai had prided itself on how closely its clinicians and scientists worked together, on the floors, in the labs, and bridging what is too often the clinical-research divide. Those collaborations rose to an unprecedented level, an all-hands-on-deck urgency to treat, discover, and remain safe amid a highly contagious virus about which so little was known. "Mount Sinai's culture was abundantly clear," said James S. Tisch, co-chair of the Boards of Trustees. "These were people who liked each other, respected each other, and were accustomed to working collaboratively and collegially."

Across Mount Sinai's hospitals and labs, workflows were streamlined, teamwork choreographed, and hierarchies flattened, empowering leadership at all levels. People worked outside their scope and were redeployed outside their own areas—often outside their own hospitals—to pitch in wherever, whenever, and however needed. Researchers and clinicians shared observations, insights, and discoveries in real time to advance testing and treatment however and with whatever they could. Data scientists were an important part of this team, making sure clinicians and researchers had up-to-date real-world evidence to inform their actions against a fast-changing illness. And, as these pages demonstrate again and again, the global collaboration of Mount Sinai's normally collaborative research enterprise was magnified, as scientists widely shared insights, resources, and discoveries in their urgent pursuit of answers.

There was also an unusual degree of collaboration among New York City's academic medical centers, including frequent conversations among overall health systems leadership, as well as leaders in emergency medicine, pathology, medical education, nursing, and other areas. "It's a story of these unbelievably competitive health care systems in New York City, which do not play nice very often, getting together weekly and strategizing together," said Brendan Carr, Mount Sinai's chair of emergency medicine. "It became a forum for collaboration across the city to solve a problem together." Dr. Carr, whose background is in preparedness and who has been actively involved in much after-action planning, said he hoped that the health systems could consolidate those gains and get even better about sharing supply-and-demand data, so they could navigate together in the face of the next exogenous shocks.

Mount Sinai also played a key role in the kind of collaboration that preparedness leaders like Dr. Carr believe is the backbone of a resilient, future-looking health care system: Public-private partnerships. Mount Sinai's clinicians, scientists, and administrators collaborated early and often with city, state, and national officials, including speaking and working closely with the likes of the NIH, CDC, and HHS. These conversations and collaborations are not out of the ordinary. They are central to how scientific and medical advancements are shared and implemented. During the pandemic, which spread in waves from region to region, these partnerships were more crucial than ever, essential to understanding and sharing best practices when so little was known and so much was at stake.

Gaining considerable knowledge and experience very early on in the pandemic, Mount Sinai experts in anticoagulation, convalescent plasma, infection prevention and PPE preservation, emergency planning, critical care pathways, palliative care, neurology challenges, wellness, and equity, among other areas, were tapped to share their insights with colleagues across the nation and the world in a number of public-private partnerships. This included regular appearances in a virtual peer-to-peer educational series called Project ECHO COVID-19 Clinical Rounds, spearheaded by the HHS Office of the Assistant Secretary for Preparedness and Response, and participation with the Healthcare Leadership Council, which gave voice to the industry's experiences and challenges in responding to the pandemic.

After-action reports have called for strategically building and strengthening such public-private partnerships—recognizing these are the alliances that have the expertise, resources, and reach needed to tackle a public health emergency of such complexity and magnitude, one that penetrates the private health care system so deeply and broadly.

⁑

ACCELERATING THE PACE OF MEDICINE AND SCIENCE

'I'm not even exaggerating. The information flows
were that rapid.'

FUELED BY URGENT NEED and powered by unprecedented collaboration, the pandemic fundamentally changed health care's axis of time. There was, essentially, the way time passed before the pandemic—often glacially, through oceans of red tape and seas of *how things have always been done*—and how time passed during the pandemic. Things that used to take months or years now took days or weeks.

That included forging the Mount Sinai Health System itself. Integrating piece by piece, strategy by strategy, since its founding in 2013, the health system in March 2020 began to move at pandemic speed in thinking and acting as a single entity. When the health system's operational leadership came to understand the depths of the COVID-19 crisis at Mount Sinai Brooklyn, it was the next morning at six-thirty that interim leaders, described by clinicians there as "the cavalry," walked through the doors to bring relief to an overwhelmed staff. And when one of those overworked staff members finally received relief in the form of outside nurses specializing in anesthesiology, he oriented them to the hospital's equipment and procedures in hours rather than weeks. So, finally, he could go home to sleep.

Collaboration enabled Mount Sinai to mobilize its medicine, science, and operations at the accelerated pace that the pandemic demanded. Interviews for this book found countless examples. A protocol for anticoagulants that was built from the ground up and rolled out to all Mount Sinai hospitals in less than two weeks. Integrating data systems across an enormous health system in weeks rather than years. Developing a quantitative antibody test shortly after the SARS-CoV-2 sequence was released, and speeding its transition to clinical use in the midst of Mount Sinai's first wave. Working around the clock to translate the potential benefits of convalescent plasma to desperate patients in a matter of days. This was the way medicine and science operated during the early part of the pandemic, often under the rubric of Emergency Use Authorization—a designation that also extended to the pharmaceutical industry's four global vaccines, developed and distributed in record time. For its part, telehealth had been making incremental progress around the edges of health care for years. Then, in days, it became an essential part of health care delivery (more on that next).

Working at such a pace demanded agility and an open mind in the face of constant change and great unknowns. Recalled Jonathan

Nover, Mount Sinai Queens' emergency department nursing senior director, "We would have a huddle at 7 a.m. with new information we literally just received at 6 a.m. Then at 10 a.m. it would change, and we would re-huddle. Same at 5 p.m. I'm not even exaggerating. The information flows were that rapid."

The hope is that the health care system and the scientific research enterprise—driven by responsiveness to global clamor—will remain better paced for progress and will hold onto the hard-won efficiencies detailed in these pages.

⁂

INNOVATING NEW CARE DELIVERY MODELS
'I don't think we're ever going back to "normal"'

UNDER DURESS, the health care system built into its future, creating flexible care delivery models, spaces that can surge up or ramp down, and an elevated role for the patient as an essential partner in understanding and treating disease. Many exigent strategies—new ways of working born of necessity—have been chronicled here, such as redeploying staff, expanding into nontraditional spaces, and double-bedding ICUs.

Mount Sinai, and health care systems across the country, also increasingly turned to telemedicine, which many see as an advance that is here to stay. "Now that people have tasted the wine, they're not coming back to water," said Dr. Carr, referring to the elixir that is the convenience of seeing a clinician without having to travel or sit in a waiting room. "I don't think we're ever going back to 'normal,' in the way people get their health care. You used to have very limited options. You go to your doctor's office, or you go to the emergency department." More recently, he said, urgent care had been added to the mix. But health systems innovated further during the pandemic, with the transformational rise in telehealth, and are now in the process of assessing value to determine which care delivery models are right for how people live and seek care today, in and beyond a pandemic.

Another takeaway from delivery of care during the pandemic was the central importance of listening to the patient, something health care has been seeking (or professing) to do in recent years, but the trend was greatly amplified by the global spread of a novel virus. Acute COVID and most especially chronic COVID have, in many ways, been defined by *experience* as much as by medicine and science. And it was only by both carefully observing and closely listening to patients that clinicians could truly determine the full contours of an illness never before seen. "Clinicians have part of the picture, but they don't have the whole picture," said Girish Nadkarni, a physician-scientist particularly attuned to information of all kinds and how it can illuminate care. "Data scientists have part of the puzzle. But then it's patients who can actually tell you what's most important to them. Without patients, you'd be missing a big, big part of the puzzle."

BUILDING RESILIENCE

'How do we build on this moment?'

AMONG THE FAILURES the 9/11 Commission cited during that crisis twenty years earlier was the failure of imagination. The same could be said of the health care system in the face of a global pandemic. The failure of imagination was not a wholesale one. Indeed, many people I spoke with have been preparing for a large-scale threat, even a viral pandemic, for years. Mount Sinai's microbiology department, in particular. It had an infrastructure, a mindset, and deep experience to quickly advance its pandemic research, and Mount Sinai scientists had among the earliest salient findings on SARS-CoV-2 antibody response and phylogenetic analysis, among other insights.

But it quickly became clear in New York and, cascadingly, across the country that the U.S. health care system would have a hard time with an overwhelming threat to human life that was both precipitous and long-lasting. "We have a standing army, navy, and air force even when we're not at war," said Mount Sinai's CEO, Kenneth Davis.

"We're paying a lot for that defense so that if we should be attacked, we're in place. Well, now the bugs and the viruses are going to attack us. And are we ready? Are we prepared? Do we have that standing army? No, we don't. What we have is a health care system that works as frugally as it can because it's under such incredible pressure around its revenues and expenses."

Dr. Davis and other health care leaders have decried American health care's mandate to ever-lower margins, a just-in-time setup that leaves organizations—and the industry as a whole—ill-prepared to ramp up systems, space, staff, and stuff when confronted with capacious exigent need, as in a pandemic. In an Op-Ed in *The Hill*, written a year after COVID-19 surfaced in New York, Drs. Davis and Carr implored the nation to invest in health care preparedness, in making sure that a network of hospitals is prepared to increase capacity "on a dime," including capacity of space and trained staff. The future, Drs. Davis and Carr wrote, demands "a paradigm shift in how we think about the intersection of routine care, unscheduled care, and the health of the populations we serve."

During its spring surge—a surge that many hospitals and health systems across the country continue to undergo as of this writing— Mount Sinai experienced a global scramble for personal protective equipment and life-saving ventilators amid broken supply chains. It faced a supply-and-demand mismatch that prompted exigent, even harrowing, decisions—double-bedding ICU rooms, building a field hospital, jury-rigging secure, if loud, negative-pressure rooms to keep patients and staff safe. The health system reimagined staffing on a massive scale, repositioning health care workers by the hundreds and redoubling efforts to support their fast-emerging mental health needs.

Many—including me, in these pages—have hailed the courage, collaboration, and sheer ingenuity that raised a field hospital in Central Park, fashioned ventilators out of home sleep-apnea devices, flew an N95 mask airlift out of China. That quickly stood up an additional high-level biocontainment space to accommodate accelerating research. That prompted health care workers, during long, grave, and graveyard shifts, to occupy the far reaches of human compassion and competence to care for an unprecedented number of patients struggling between life and death.

But there's another side to it. The fact that one of the finest health systems in the world had to resort to heroic moves to surmount the pandemic reveals how far the health care system needs to go to be ready for the next one. In September 2021, almost a year and a half after the pandemic first swept through New York, more than ten states were experiencing the highest hospitalization rates of the entire pandemic (one in four hospitals reported ICUs more than 95 percent full). Field hospitals were springing up in parking garages across the South.

How, then, to consolidate learnings from the exigent capacity building—of physical spaces, of essential resources, of desperately needed health care workers—done under the full weight and urgency of the pandemic surge?

The best defense begins with a good offense. "All your characteristics—good, bad, and indifferent—come out during a crisis," said Art Gianelli, president of Mount Sinai Morningside and chief transformation officer for the health system. "So invest your capital broadly in your organization, in your culture, teams, data sources, systems and processes, work and workflow improvements. Then you draw down on those investments in a crisis."

Pre-pandemic, Mount Sinai was as well positioned as any organization could be for what was to come. It was well capitalized, with a great deal of expertise and excellence in medicine and science, and a culture of innovation and collaboration. And it was a health *system*, a strategically broad-based network of hospitals integrated with a medical school. It became clear in March and April 2020 that if Mount Sinai's smaller community hospitals had been stand-alone entities, they would have sunk under the weight of too many acutely ill patients, too little staff, and inadequate connection to up-to-the-minute therapeutic protocols. Catalyzed during the first wave, Mount Sinai increasingly thought, acted, and communicated as a unified entity, proactively distributing people, resources, and therapeutic protocols where needed, across a large footprint. "All of a sudden, everything that was ordered for any single hospital wasn't going to that hospital. It was going central and was deployed where it was needed most," said System President and COO Margaret Pastuszko, reflecting on that operational pivot. "I could give you a thousand examples."

An integrated health care system makes flexibility possible, and flexibility is an essential part of preparedness—extending to spaces, staff, and stuff. Mount Sinai, among many other health care systems, built out an enormous number of spaces during the surge, creating negative-pressure rooms and refitting spaces as intensive care units, and will aim to retain that flexibility into the future. "Some modifications we've made around the hospital we probably won't take down" after the COVID surge, Lucy Xenophon, chief transformation officer at Mount Sinai Morningside, told The Lens podcast, enumerating lessons learned from the first wave. "We've learned something about new spaces we're building, and we're going to—to the extent possible—make them flexible spaces, so we can bring in ICU patients if need were to arise."

Flexibility was a common theme as Mount Sinai leaders redeployed health care workers from unit to unit, hospital to hospital, employing a team-based model of care that will surely remain central to future planning. Mount Sinai also went to great lengths to build up flexibility in sourcing and in the supply chain, so health care doesn't fall victim to the comprehensive slowdowns that delayed or derailed resources during 2020 and into 2021. Flexibility, too, extends to new care delivery models, such as telehealth, and to ensuring that spaces, staffing, and protective equipment allow for hospital visitors, avoiding in the future the additional layers of grief wrought by a no-visitors policy.

Before the pandemic, "flexibility" and "health care" might not have lived easily together in a sentence. But, Dr. Boal pointed out, flexibility is actually at the heart of evidence-based medicine—and in the hearts of those trained to practice it. "Learning from our mistakes, trying new things, evolving along the way ... is really what it comes down to," he said. "The good news is that in many ways, that's a hallmark of the scientific method. That's what we're all trained in. We can ... look at the facts and draw insights ... and change what we do. And not get overwhelmed by it."

Among its many preparedness efforts, Mount Sinai has launched a Center for Healthcare Readiness to advance research, policy, education, and action to, as its vision states, "ensure the healthcare system can meet the needs of our patient populations." One of its core competencies is bridging frontline medical providers and system scientists, including with aggressive data collection and deployment critical to a better prepared future. "We were changing all of our processes, and we needed to measure the ripple effect of those changes so we could improve," said Dr. Carr, citing, by way of example, measuring throughput in the emergency department, seeing where and when bottlenecks occurred. "That's what it means to be a learning health system. You have to both fly the plane and build it. So as you go along, you're learning, you're learning, you're learning. We are always looking at our delivery system and our outcomes, analyzing the data, borrowing research tools to drive clinical care and operations in a rapid-cycle way."

Recently, Dr. Carr explained, Mount Sinai gathered data from its spring 2020 surge to help the U.S. Department of Defense better benchmark the upper limits of the private health care system's capacity—something that had previously been a theoretical exercise. "Before COVID, no one had pushed themselves to the limit," said Dr. Carr.

The pandemic changed that. Now, Mount Sinai and other private hospitals were able to create those benchmarks as an important pillar in the DOD's emergency planning. "That's a lasting gift that we give them," said Dr. Carr, "a guidepost for the nation to understand the capacity within the civilian health care system."

RESILIENCE ALSO INCLUDES deep and sustained attention to health care workers' mental health. Studies at Mount Sinai and elsewhere have shown that when workers feel supported by their employers, they report more resilience. Mount Sinai codified that support early in the pandemic with, among other endeavors, its Center for Stress, Resilience, and Personal Growth (see Chapter 13). Other elements of resilience-building were in evidence during the pandemic by the very nature of the work, with employees uniting in common mission, feeling empowered to lead at all levels, and experiencing—indeed, relying upon—a sense of collaboration and camaraderie. As Barbara Murphy, the system's chair of medicine who was responsible for organizing much of the clinical staffing redeployment, said, "It was an amazing time, if it wasn't so awful."

Dr. Carr began a recent conversation about looking back on and looking forward from the pandemic this way: "I don't know how you talk about how broken people are a year and a half in." These pages have chronicled health care workers' suffering during, and rising to, the most challenging times in their professional lives, without even the small niceties of the day. No leaning on a shoulder, chatting with a colleague in the hallway, or even sipping a cup of coffee at work.

People are leaving health care professions, or thinking seriously about it. A year after the first wave hit New York City, a Washington Post-Kaiser Family Foundation survey found that almost 30 percent of health care workers have considered leaving the field following the stress of COVID. A study in a *Lancet* open-access journal in May 2021 found that almost half of health care workers reported feeling burnout, with women, people of color, and those in allied health professions (as compared to physicians) suffering disproportionately.

At the same time, applications to medical schools were up a record double-digit percentage in 2021, including 26 percent to Mount Sinai. Medical students, many of whom came of professional age during the pandemic, are a fulcrum between the present and future of the health care system. Charles Sanky was in his final year of Mount Sinai's medical school during the pandemic before starting his residency in emergency medicine at Mount Sinai in 2021. Graduating with degrees in medicine, business, and public health, he is committed to creating the systems-level changes he would like to see. "How do we build on this moment?" asked Dr. Sanky. "I'd like to reimagine health system design, health equity, and health care readiness, so that everything we do—every single workflow, every single protocol—makes us ready for what happens next. People don't want to be called heroes. They want a better health care system."

After nineteen months of a global pandemic, the health care system and health care workers are reeling—still standing but forever changed, in ways large and small, many of which have been written about here. In one workaday example, nurses at Mount Sinai Queens found it hard to return to a simple pre-pandemic protocol after the initial first wave had receded: leaving patient doors open. Before COVID, an open patient door was the preferred mode, for both ease of clinical oversight and greater patient satisfaction. But habits forged in battle can be hard to break. The seal on those doors—so negative pressure could collect the virus's contagion—had for months been the barrier between risk and relative safety.

We have all been navigating our way between risk and relative safety for a year and a half. As I write this, on September 15, 2021, statistics showed that 1 in 500 Americans had died of COVID-19.

It's hard to know what note to end on. One of hope, of peril? Of exhaustion, or resolve? Diagnosis has improved and become more accessible, as has treatment. Depending on the severity of illness, therapies include monoclonal antibodies, remdesivir, and dexamethasone. And prevention—those vaccines! When they first came out at the end of 2020, within a year of the virus's first appearing in humans, they promised to change the trajectory of the pandemic. And in many ways they have. But access and uptake have been stubbornly slow and inconsistent. The Delta variant has been accelerating spread, even in vaccinated people. The latter part of 2021, as noted at the beginning of the book, found the world in a race between vaccines and variants.

Progress is steady, but hope is checkered.

CHAPTER

16

GOING HOME

'I was reborn'

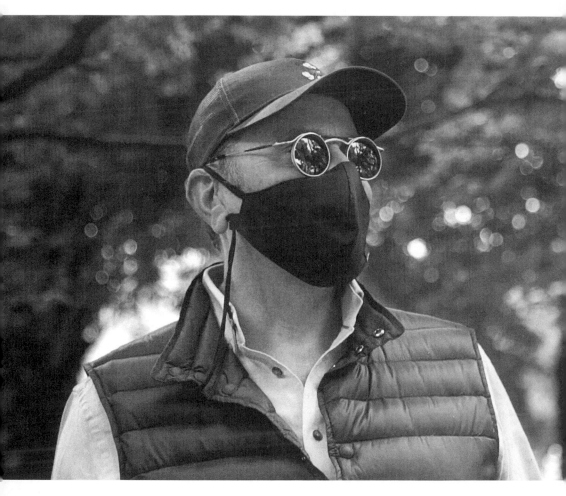

Rodrigo Saval, Mount Sinai's first COVID-19 inpatient, had a profound effect on the team who cared for him over his long hospital stay.

APRIL 12, 2020—On Easter Sunday, Rodrigo Saval woke up. He opened his eyes and saw people outside his ICU room, applauding. He asked himself, *Who are these people? Where am I?* He touched his face and felt something unfamiliar: forty days' growth of a beard. *Oh my God, how long has it been?* he wondered.

The Mount Sinai Health System was still near its peak COVID population, caring for more than 1,600 COVID patients.

Clinicians filled Mr. Saval in on all that had happened, including intubation and a tracheostomy, which was still in place. He learned that he had been dialyzed because his kidneys stopped working and that he had suffered from blood clots and was on a regimen of blood thinners.

When his care providers sought to connect him to his family and friends, he felt like Rip Van Winkle after sleeping through time. "They asked me, 'Do you want to Zoom with your family?'" he recounted. "And I said, 'What's a Zoom?' On March the third, nobody was talking about Zooming." He had been intubated when New Yorkers were still gathering in person, hugging, traveling, and going to work, school, restaurants, and theater. Since then, the technology platform had replaced in-person everything: meetings, classes, holiday gatherings, and, in evidence across Mount Sinai, patient visits by family and friends. Mr. Saval couldn't speak because of the tracheostomy, but he was overcome with emotion seeing his family for the first time in more than a month.

He was soon moved to a step-down unit, but his role as a talisman continued. Care providers would visit his room because of his engaging personality, because he had been the first patient, and because he had endured. Someone from palliative care visited him to let him know that when he had been near death, she had come to hold his hand. She came back a couple of times once he was on the mend. The third time, as Mr. Saval tells it, he asked her, "Am I dying?" No, no, she answered. She just liked visiting him. As he did with many of his care providers, Mr. Saval remained in touch with her well after his discharge.

At the end of April, Mount Sinai's COVID patient population had begun to drop below a thousand for the first time in a month. On April 29, it was 866—a number that would no longer include Mr. Saval. That day, the health system's first COVID inpatient left the hospital as Mount Sinai West's 500th discharge. He headed back to his apartment with a prescription for home health care and physical therapy arranged by a Mount Sinai social worker. Scores of health care workers lined hospital corridors, cheering and clapping in all their PPE. The Beatles' "Here Comes the Sun"—the farewell anthem initiated at Mount Sinai South Nassau and adopted by many other Mount Sinai hospitals—soared through the lobby. Mr. Saval's wheelchair was festooned with balloons.

"We needed this win," said Jennie Drexler, nurse manager in the ICU, who devoted much time and care to Mr. Saval.

Joseph Mathew, the ICU director, was partly responsible for the large crowd bidding Mr. Saval farewell. Upon learning of the impending discharge, Dr. Mathew went back into the patient's medical record and was reminded of the many people along the way who provided more than fifty days of life-saving care. He alerted them to the discharge. The ED team, ED techs, respiratory therapists, nurses, environmental services, the anesthesiologist who intubated Mr. Saval, palliative care. The physical and respiratory therapists who treated him after he left the ICU for the medical floor. Administrative and clinical leadership were there, too.

"The main thing that this pandemic taught us is, really, it takes a village to get somebody better," said Dr. Mathew. "Everyone who was involved in his care came out to greet him. It's a nice testament to the idea that we need team-based care—and not just during COVID—to get people better."

For Mr. Saval's part, he had weeks' worth of nightmares to process now that he was awake. He hadn't been in physical pain, he said, but just under the surface of consciousness he had been trying to make sense of why he couldn't move and people were in and out of the room probing him. At the same time, he said, he felt comforted. "I never felt alone, that I was going to die alone."

His near-death experiences came back to him in a flood of peace a couple months later when he traveled home to Chile for his father's death from a brain tumor. "As he was dying, I had this flashback that I had been there, at the place where he was, suspended in the air," Mr. Saval recalled, growing emotional. "Everything was white. It was such a wonderful feeling that I could not describe. More than being in love, more than joy. Peace. It was something that we human beings don't go through until we are at that stage where actually we are dying."

COVID, he said, did not exactly change his view of life. It changed his view of death.

LARRY KELLY opened his eyes on Easter Sunday, too, but he would remain on a ventilator until May and would be moved to Mount Sinai Beth Israel for intensive rehabilitation. Clinicians were initially concerned about his cognitive function, as he had been on a ventilator for fifty-one days. But, slowly, surely, he got better. He went to a skilled nursing facility at the end of May, and, on July 22, one hundred twenty-eight days after he was first hospitalized, he went home, earning him the nickname "Miracle Larry."

Jessica Montanaro, the nurse who welcomed him to the ICU and told him she'd help him breathe, who stood by his room with his wife, Dawn, to have what the nurse thought was an end-of-life conversation but his wife thought was a do-everything-you-can conversation, now got to see Mr. Kelly go home. "He has a long road, and I'm sure it's been extremely emotional, but he's got his life back," Ms. Montanaro said, adding that they have stayed in touch. "We call each other family. We say we're bonded for life."

In November, Mr. Kelly returned to Mount Sinai via Zoom to speak, alongside his wife, to Mirna Mohanraj's class of pulmonary critical care fellows. As an ICU survivor, he had valuable lessons for the fellows. For one thing, he told them he was aware of much more than it might have seemed, and he'd once heard a negative conversation about his prognosis. "There's so much value in remembering that we can keep the medical conversations out of the room and ensure that we always are speaking to the patient as if they're awake and with us in the room," said Dr. Mohanraj.

Even in a coma, Mr. Kelly had felt the balm of company and the sting of isolation. "They like us to talk to them and spend time with them outside of our routine care," Dr. Mohanraj said, noting that she has heard similar sentiments from other former ICU patients. "With our non-COVID patients, we do pop in all the time and chat. But that was tough with COVID. The burden of COVID was that our time was so limited, and patients felt that limitation."

Back in Chile for Thanksgiving 2020, Rodrigo Saval introduced his local friends and family, by video, to Dr. Mathew and various members of the team at Mount Sinai whom the Chilean credited for saving his life. "Dr. Mathew said to my family that I could feel I have family at Mount Sinai," said Mr. Saval. He was eagerly awaiting the COVID-19 vaccine so he could get back to visit that newfound family, get back to New York.

"I was reborn there," he said.

ACKNOWLEDGEMENTS

THANK YOU to the doctors, nurses, scientists, administrators, staff, students, and patients of Mount Sinai for their extraordinary generosity—with all else they were doing—in sharing their stories so passionately and eloquently. Thank you to Marc Kaplan, Mark Goldberg, Alan Flippen, Leslie Kirschenbaum, and Cathy Clarke for keen editorial and visual insights from beginning to end. And thank you to my family for patience, support, and inspiration, in and out of quarantine.

END NOTES

MOST OF THE INFORMATION in this book comes from interviews with more than one hundred people affiliated with Mount Sinai, including clinicians, researchers, administrators, staff, hospital and medical school leadership, and patients. The end notes below detail additional sourcing information, as well as further notes and context.

AUTHOR'S NOTE

1 *global death toll:* "COVID-19 Map." Johns Hopkins Coronavirus Resource Center, coronavirus.jhu.edu/map.html.

1 *began on December 15:* "Mount Sinai Employees Explain Why They Were Excited to Receive the New COVID-19 Vaccine." *Mount Sinai Today,* 18 Dec. 2020, health. mountsinai.org/blog/mount-sinai-employees-explain-why-they-were-excited-to-receive-the-new-covid-19-vaccine/.

CHAPTER 1

14 *the husband tested negative:* The husband later tested positive for robust COVID antibodies and went on to become a convalescent plasma donor.

14 *"Community spread is going to be real":* McKinley, Jesse, and Joseph Goldstein. "Coronavirus Outbreak Will Spread in New York City, Officials Warn." *The New York Times,* 2 Mar. 2020, www.nytimes.com/2020/03/02/nyregion/ coronavirus-new-york.html.

15 *a second case of COVID-19:* Goldstein, Joseph, and Jesse McKinley. "Second Case of Coronavirus in N.Y. Sets off Search for Others Exposed." *The New York Times,* 3 Mar. 2020, www.nytimes.com/2020/03/03/nyregion/coronavi-rus-new-york-state.html.

15 *more than 111 million people across the globe:* "COVID-19 Map." Johns Hopkins Coronavirus Resource Center.

15 *203,000 people testing COVID-positive in New York:* "COVID-19 Outbreak -

New York City, February 29–June 1, 2020." Centers for Disease Control and Prevention, 17 Dec. 2020, www.cdc.gov/mmwr/volmes/69/wr/mm6946a2.htm.

16 *20 percent to 30 percent:* Richardson, Safiya, et al. "Presenting Characteristics, Comorbidities, and Outcomes among 5700 Patients Hospitalized With COVID-19 in the New York City Area." *JAMA,* vol. 323, no. 20, 22 Apr. 2020, p. 2052, doi:10.1001/jama.2020.6775. *See also:* Paranjpe, Ishan, et al. "Retrospective Cohort Study of Clinical Characteristics of 2199 Hospitalised Patients With COVID-19 in New York City." *BMJ Open,* vol. 10, no. 11, 27 Nov. 2020, doi:10.1136/bmjopen-2020-040736.

16 *Twenty-one people aboard a cruise ship:* Rodriguez, Olga R. "21 Positive for Coronavirus on Cruise Ship off California." Associated Press, 7 Mar. 2020, apnews.com/article/nv-state-wire-wa-state-wire-ri-state-wire-co-state-wire-virus-outbreak-61a4efa966c02cbda9584f7266b99802.

16 *Intensivists like Dr. Mathew:* Dr. Roopa Kohli-Seth, director of Mount Sinai's Institute for Critical Care, gave a concise description of an intensivist. "So, you want to know who is an intensivist? They should be able to save a patient's life. They have to be quick-witted and able to multitask, manage a patient, intubate, do vascular access, have knowledge of all the medications, paralytics, antibiotics, and have current knowledge of what things save lives."

17 *Raymonde Jean:* YouTube, Mount Sinai West, 2 May 2020, www.youtube.com/?gl=NL.

18 *Krystina Woods:* YouTube, Mount Sinai West, 2 May 2020, www.youtube.com/watch?v=tGfjNXTk8lo.

CHAPTER 2

23 *blocks one of the key enzymes:* "Final Report Confirms Remdesivir Benefits for COVID-19." U.S. Department of Health and Human Services, National Institutes of Health, 27 Oct. 2020, www.nih.gov/news-events/nih-research-matters/final-report-confirms-remdesivir-benefits-covid-19.

23 *While the drug was not yet FDA-approved:* Remdesivir would go on to receive Emergency Use Authorization from the FDA on May 1 and would come to be one of the most promising treatments throughout 2020, including use in a three-part therapeutic cocktail delivered to President Trump in October. *See:* "Coronavirus (COVID-19) Update: FDA Issues Emergency Use Authorization for Potential Covid-19 Treatment." U.S. Food and Drug Administration, 1 May 2020, www.fda.gov/news-events/press-announcements/coronavirus-covid-19-update-fda-issues-emergency-use-authorization-potential-covid-19-treatment.

23 *expanded access:* "Expanded Access." U.S. Food and Drug Administration, www.fda.gov/news-events/public-health-focus/expanded-access.

25 *cytokine storm:* Del Valle, Diane Marie, et al. "An Inflammatory Cytokine Signature Predicts COVID-19 Severity and Survival." *Nature Medicine,* vol. 26, no. 10, 24 Aug. 2020, pp. 1636–1643, doi:10.1038/s41591-020-1051-9.

26 *Rafael Miranda:* "Transporters Show Great Agility, Empathy, and Teamwork in Uncertain Times." *Mount Sinai Today,* 14 May 2020, health.mountsinai.org/blog/transporters-show-great-agility-empathy-and-teamwork-in-uncertain-times/.

26 *fit-tested:* Per Occupational Safety and Health Administration (OSHA) requirements: "The test shall not be conducted if there is any hair growth between the

skin and the facepiece sealing surface, such as stubble beard growth, beard, mustache or sideburns [that] cross the respirator sealing surface." *See:* "1910.134 App A - Fit Testing Procedures (Mandatory). Occupational Safety and Health Administration." United States Department of Labor, OSHA, www.osha.gov/laws-regs/regulations/standardnumber/1910/1910.134AppA.

27 *Rubiela Guzman:* Lindsay Lyon. "Treating Patients amid Covid-19's Peak in New York: 'All of Us Feel Forever Changed.'" *U.S. News & World Report,* 28 May 2020, health.usnews.com/hospital-heroes/articles/covid-19-in-hard-hit-new-york-city-a-massive-team-effort-at-mount-sinai.

28 *Tedros Adhanom Ghebreyesus:* @DrTedros (Tedros Adhanom Ghebreyesus), ".@WHO Is Deeply Concerned by the Alarming Levels of the #Coronavirus Spread, Severity & Inaction, & Expects to See the Number of Cases, Deaths & Affected Countries Climb Even Higher. Therefore, We Made the Assessment THAT #covid19 Can Be Characterized as a Pandemic." Twitter, 11 Mar. 2020, twitter.com/drtedros/status/1237800182235922434?lang=en.

29 *the journal Science:* Gonzalez-Reiche, Ana S., et al. "Introductions and Early Spread of SARS-CoV-2 in the New York City Area." *Science,* vol. 369, no. 6501, 17 July 2020, pp. 297–301, doi:10.1126/science.abc1917.

30 *pivotal autopsy study:* Bryce, Clare, et al. "Pathophysiology of SARS-CoV-2: The Mount Sinai COVID-19 Autopsy Experience." *Modern Pathology,* vol. 34, no. 8, 1 Apr. 2021, pp. 1456–1467, doi:10.1038/s41379-021-00793-y. (preprinted online May 2020)

31 *Two hundred twenty-two COVID patients:* This and all subsequent patient census figures, unless otherwise noted, refer to retrospective data culled from the Mount Sinai Health System's electronic health record. These figures may differ from those cited by hospital leaders in the middle of the pandemic, which often drew from real-time data reported at daily huddles and prospective-modeling data delivered frequently to clinical and operational leaders.

31 *Madeline Hernandez:* "National Nurses Week: The Givers." Mount Sinai Health System, Road to Resilience Podcast, 8 May 2020, www.mountsinai.org/about/newsroom/podcasts/road-resilience/the-givers.

34 *whose husband would go on to contract COVID:* Ms. Montanaro wrote in a March 29, 2020, email to hospital president Arthur Gianelli, "Pretty sure my husband is positive for corona (official testing appointment tomorrow). But I'm coming in every day to fight this because there's not much I can do for him while I have him quarantined in our house. I feel and have felt fine. I haven't seen him in so long because I was working feverishly at the hospital and he was working to keep his business afloat and when he started not feeling well, I quarantined him right away. I have my children taking care of him through the door...my 10-year-old (I dubbed her "Dr. Montanaro") has to feed him certain amount of fluids every day (per mommy). I nurse him through FaceTime while I'm at the hospital. I have him on continuous oxygen-saturation monitoring on the third floor of our house and I am in close contact with his doctors and ours about his condition."

35 *David Van De Carr:* "From the Frontlines." YouTube, Mount Sinai Health System, 11 May 2020, www.youtube.com/watch?v=dsFtYwpIOHQ.

40 *via Facetime and Zoom:* Serendipitously, as part of its regular review and revision of vendors, Mount Sinai switched its telecommunications in January 2020 from a well-known platform, Arkadin, to a lesser-known platform called Zoom. That meant that Mount Sinai had already switched over to the new platform's internet

and telephone capabilities by the time Zoom seemed to take over the world in spring 2020, with so many people working from home and families and friends distancing from one another.

41 *Valerie Burgos-Kneeland:* "National Nurses Week: The Givers." Mount Sinai Health System, Road to Resilience Podcast, 8 May 2020, www.mountsinai.org/about/newsroom/podcasts/road-resilience/the-givers.

41 *Camille Davis:* Wilber, Del Quentin. "'We Are Used to Death ... but Not on This Scale': An Oral History of the Coronavirus Crisis." *Los Angeles Times,* 21 Apr. 2020, www.latimes.com/world-nation/story/2020-04-21/coronavirus-oral-history.

43 *Jennifer Jaromahum:* Ms. Jaromahum left Mount Sinai in 2021, after shepherding Mount Sinai West's nursing team through the worst of the pandemic in 2020.

47 *she said after her brief recharge:* "From the Frontlines: Recharge Room." Facebook, The Mount Sinai Hospital, 15 Apr. 2020, www.facebook.com/watch/?v=653677641843277.

48 *she told Wired magazine:* Roberts, LaVonne. "These Recharge Rooms Are Helping Health Care Workers Cope." *Wired,* 21 Jan. 2021, www.wired.com/story/covid-recharge-rooms-health-care-front-line/.

49 *nearly 40 percent of health care workers:* Feingold, Jordyn H., et al. "Psychological Impact of the COVID-19 Pandemic on Frontline Health Care Workers during the Pandemic Surge in New York City." *Chronic Stress,* vol. 5, 1 Feb. 2021, p. 247054702097789, doi:10.1177/2470547020977891.

50 *Maria Duenas:* from the Mount Sinai Archives project, COVID Memories.

52 *End of Life Companion Program:* "Volunteering Their Time and Hearts to Share a Heavy Burden." *Mount Sinai Today,* 15 May 2020, health.mountsinai.org/blog/volunteering-their-time-and-hearts-to-share-a-heavy-burden/.

52 *Amparo Sullivan encouraged her colleagues:* "Mount Sinai Queens Nurses Share Memories With COVID-19 Patients' Survivors." *Mount Sinai Today,* 16 July 2020, health.mountsinai.org/blog/mount-sinai-queens-nurses-share-memories-with-covid-19-patients-survivors/.

CHAPTER 3

56 *Emil von Behring:* Mock, Jillian. "The Peculiar 100-plus-Year History of Convalescent Plasma." *Smithsonian Magazine,* 1 Sept. 2020, www.smithsonianmag.com/science-nature/peculiar-100-plus-year-history-convalescent-plasma-180975683/.

56 *his assay was the first:* Amanat, Fatima, et al. "A Serological Assay to Detect SARS-CoV-2 Seroconversion in Humans." *Nature Medicine,* vol. 26, no. 7, 12 May 2020, pp. 1033–1036, doi:10.1038/s41591-020-0913-5.

57 *went a little viral:* Grady, Denise. "Blood Plasma from Survivors Will Be given to Coronavirus Patients." *The New York Times,* 26 Mar. 2020, www.nytimes.com/2020/03/26/health/plasma-coronavirus-treatment.html.

58 *Riemer told NBC News:* Ferguson, Conor, et al. "Plasma Treatment Being Tested in New York May Be Coronavirus 'Game Changer.'" NBCNews.com, 8 Apr. 2020, www.nbcnews.com/health/health-news/plasma-treatment-

being-tested-new-york-may-be-coronavirus-gamechanger-n1178436.

59 *Claudia Garcenot:* Silman, Anna. "Diary of a Hospital: 'Now I Know the Horror That They're Living.'" *New York Magazine,* 24 Apr. 2020, nymag.com/intelligencer/2020/04/coronavirus-nyc-nurse-isolation.html.

60 *Jennifer Woodard:* Mount Sinai South Nassau newsletter, Vol. 1. Issue 10.

60 *In results published in Nature Medicine:* Liu, Sean T., et al. "Convalescent Plasma Treatment of Severe COVID-19: A Propensity Score–Matched Control Study." *Nature Medicine,* vol. 26, no. 11, 15 Sept. 2020, pp. 1708–1713, doi:10.1038/s41591-020-1088-9.

61 *in late March and early April:* The use of convalescent plasma—whether as a part of an eIND program or, later, clinical trials—tapered off for lack of evidence in the months that followed. In February 2021, the NIH halted a multisite (not including Mount Sinai) clinical trial of convalescent plasma in non-severe emergency department patients, noting that the treatment was not likely to confer benefits. *See:* "NIH Halts Trial of COVID-19 Convalescent Plasma in Emergency Department Patients with Mild Symptoms." National Institutes of Health, U.S. Department of Health and Human Services, 2 June 2021, www.nih.gov/news-events/news-releases/nih-halts-trial-covid-19-convalescent-plasma-emergency-department-patients-mild-symptoms.

"Convalescent plasma was a good treatment when we didn't know how to make virus-specific antibodies," Miriam Merad, a leading Mount Sinai immunologist, told *The Scientist Magazine.* "It was in the middle of the pandemic, and it served its purpose." *See:* Banks, Marcus A. "NIH Halts Outpatient COVID-19 Convalescent Plasma Trial." *The Scientist Magazine,* 4 Mar. 2021, www.the-scientist.com/news-opinion/nih-halts-outpatient-covid-19-convalescent-plasma-trial-68514.

61 *was better than nothing:* In the coming months, another iteration of passive immunity, monoclonal antibodies, would show signs of success in randomized controlled trials. On November 2, 2020, the FDA issued an emergency use authorization for the investigational monoclonal antibody therapy bamlanivimab, which Mount Sinai patients had access to. *See:* "Coronavirus (COVID-19) UPDATE: FDA Authorizes Monoclonal Antibody for Treatment of COVID-19." U.S. Food and Drug Administration, 9 Nov. 2020, www.fda.gov/news-events/press-announcements/coronavirus-covid-19-update-fda-authorizes-monoclonal-antibody-treatment-covid-19.

61 *medicine professor Sean Liu:* "Convalescent Plasma Is a Potentially Effective Treatment Option for Patients Hospitalized with COVID-19, According to Early Data." Mount Sinai Health System, 22 May 2020, www.mountsinai.org/about/newsroom/2020/convalescent-plasma-is-a-potentially-effective-treatment-option-for-patients-hospitalized-with-covid-19-according-to-early-data-pr.

62 *wrote the book on mechanical ventilation:* Poor, Hooman. *Basics of Mechanical Ventilation.* Springer, 2018.

62 *did not have typical pneumonias:* Poor, Hooman D., et al. "COVID-19 Critical Illness Pathophysiology Driven by Diffuse Pulmonary Thrombi and Pulmonary Endothelial Dysfunction Responsive to Thrombolysis." *Clinical and Translational Medicine,* vol. 10, no. 2, 13 May 2020, doi:10.1002/ctm2.44.

62 *major autopsy study:* Bryce, Clare, et al. "Pathophysiology of SARS-CoV-2."

62 *Dr. Mocco told NPR:* "Doctors Find Some Younger COVID-19 Patients Suffer Serious Strokes." NPR, 29 Apr. 2020, www.npr.org/2020/04/29/847732044/ doctors-find-some-younger-covid-19-patients-suffer-serious-strokes.

62 *New England Journal of Medicine:* Oxley, Thomas J., et al. "Large-Vessel Stroke as a Presenting Feature of COVID-19 in the Young." *New England Journal of Medicine,* vol. 382, no. 20, 28 Apr. 2020, doi:10.1056/nejmc2009787.

64 *John Puskas:* Edwards, Erika. "For Sickest Patients, Blood Thinners May Be Linked to Reduced COVID-19 Deaths, Study Finds." NBCNews.com, 6 May 2020, www.nbcnews.com/health/health-news/blood-thinners-may-be-linked-reduced-covid-19-deaths-study-n1201276.

67 *improved survival from COVID:* Paranjpe, Ishan, et al. "Association of Treatment Dose Anticoagulation With In-Hospital Survival Among Hospitalized Patients With COVID-19." *Journal of the American College of Cardiology,* vol. 76, no. 1, 7 July 2020, pp. 122–124, doi:10.1016/j.jacc.2020.05.001.

73 *The first set of guidelines was published:* Leibner, Evan S., et al. "Emergency Department COVID Management Policies: One Institution's Experience and Lessons Learned." *EBMedicine.net,* 28 Apr. 2020, www.ebmedicine.net/topics/infectious-disease/COVID-19/Protocols.

CHAPTER 4

79 *under one operational system:* Mount Sinai South Nassau joined more recently and was not yet fully integrated, although it benefited a great deal from resources, support, and clinical advances from the Health System; at the same time, one of the original health system hospitals, New York Eye and Ear Infirmary of Mount Sinai, was not directly involved in the pandemic response.

80 *Radio Advisory podcast:* "Mount Sinai's Chief Clinical Officer Surmounted the COVID-19 Surge. Here's His Advice for You." *Advisory Board,* Radio Advisory, 14 Aug. 2020, www.advisory.com/daily-briefing/2020/08/14/mount-sinai.

82 *mergers or acquisitions that year:* "Hospital M&A Activity Grew Slightly in 2013." *Becker's Hospital Review,* 11 Apr. 2014, www.beckershospitalreview.com/hospital-transactions-and-valuation/hospital-m-a-activity-grew-slightly-in-2013.html.

82 *said in 2015:* "Medicine 360°: A Conversation Between Kenneth L. Davis and Dennis S. Charney." *Mount Sinai Science & Medicine,* 2015, p. 2.

82 *Dean Dennis Charney:* Ibid. p. 4.

86 *as the pandemic peaked:* The Mount Sinai Health System also transfers patients from outside the system into its hospitals. During the pandemic, while most transfers occurred between system hospitals, patients from outside hospitals who needed a higher level of care were also accommodated, according to Dr. Warshaw.

CHAPTER 5

96 *oxygen we needed in the building:* Mount Sinai South Nassau underwent a similar doubling of its need, and, following the pandemic's spring peak, got to work building a new, permanent external oxygen system.

101 *Dr. Herron told New York Magazine:* Silman, Anna. "Diary of a Hospital:

The Surgical Chief Changing Soiled Bedsheets." *New York Magazine,* 29 Apr. 2020, nymag.com/intelligencer/2020/04/the-manhattan-surgeon-helping-brooklyn-coronavirus-patients.html.

CHAPTER 6

105   *transplant intensive care unit:* Transplant moved to a smaller recovery unit. Mount Sinai continued transplantation throughout COVID, with March 2020 becoming the liver transplantation program's busiest month ever, as referrals came in from other institutions that had suspended their transplant programs. *See:* "As the Nation Locked Down a Liver Transplant Team Went into Overdrive." *Mount Sinai Today,* 15 Apr. 2021, health.mountsinai.org/blog/baby-nathaniel-liver-transplant/.

105   *Which medical, surgical, and intensive care units:* The hospitals, especially the quaternary-care Mount Sinai Hospital, were still open for necessary non-COVID care. While the numbers were way down, patients still came in for cancer care, transplantation, stroke care, broken bones, and childbirth, among other care, throughout the pandemic, and the hospitals had to maintain safe spaces for those patients.

105   *Dr. Reich's recipe:* The rest of the recipe included getting the necessary "stuff" and "staff" for the space, as well as scaling up, running the recipe again and again.

109   *writing in 1864:* Bourne, William Oland. Civil War Reminiscences by Soldiers & Sailors in Central Park Hospital, NY, New York. tile.loc.gov/storage-services/service/gdc/gdccrowd/mss/mss13375/001/01/00101.txt.

110   *you run out of stuff:* Dr. Carr shared more insights into the partnership between Samaritan's Purse and Mount Sinai in a U.S. State Department Foreign Press Center briefing, April 9, 2020. https://2017-2021.state.gov/samaritans-purse-and-mount-sinai-hospitals-emergency-field-hospital-operations-in-new-yorks-central-park/index.html.

113   *reimbursement for telehealth services: See:* Adams, Katie. "A Timeline of Telehealth Support from the Federal Government during the Pandemic." *Becker's Hospital Review,* 14 Sept. 2020, www.beckershospitalreview.com/telehealth/a-timeline-of-telehealth-support-from-the-federal-government-during-the-pandemic.html.

113   *Americans would be visiting with their clinicians:* Another home-based program, one that delivered inpatient-level care at home via visiting clinicians and mobile equipment, grew in popularity during the exigencies of COVID. By letting people receive sophisticated care in the comfort of their homes, Mount Sinai's Hospitalization at Home program helped decant patients from hospital beds and meant family could be with patients.

CHAPTER 7

117   *Barbara Murphy:* Barbara Murphy, who was a world-renowned expert in kidney transplantation and was central to Mount Sinai's COVID-19 response, died in June 2021, from glioblastoma.

118   *April 17 presentation:* "Webinar April 17, 2020 - COVID-19 in the United States: Insights from Healthcare Systems." Centers for Disease Control and Prevention, 14 Apr. 2020, emergency.cdc.gov/coca/calls/2020/callinfo_041720.asp.

119 Allison Chang: "Physician Assistants Earn Praise for Supporting the Front Lines." *Mount Sinai Today,* 11 May 2020, health.mountsinai.org/blog/physician-assistants-earn-praise-for-supporting-the-front-lines/.

120 *The American Surgeon:* Vine, Anthony J. "Mount Sinai NY Surgeon on the Front Lines of the COVID-19 Pandemic in Brooklyn, NY, USA." *The American Surgeon,* vol. 86, no. 6, June 2020, pp. 567–571, doi:10.1177/0003134820924397.

121 *Long Island cardiologist Jay Dubowsky:* Dubowsky, Jay. "Away from His Clinical Home, a Physician Finds Himself among Family." *Mount Sinai Today,* 15 May 2020, health.mountsinai.org/blog/away-from-his-clinical-home-a-physician-finds-himself-among-family/.

122 *said Dr. Badhey:* "Residents Launch Nation's First ENT COVID-19 ICU." *Otolaryngology - Head and Neck Surgery,* Mount Sinai, reports.mountsinai.org/article/ent2021-03 residents-launch-nations-first-ent-intensive-care-unit.

122 *Benny Laitman described:* Laitman, Benny. "The Peak." *ENT in the Time of COVID,* 18 Apr. 2020, benlaitman.wixsite.com/website/.

123 *NEJM Catalyst:* Michelle Kang Kim, et al. "A Primer for Clinician Deployment to the Medicine Floors from an Epicenter of COVID-19." *NEJM Catalyst Innovations in Care Delivery,* 4 May 2020, catalyst.nejm.org/doi/full/10.1056/CAT.20.0180.

125 *in a New York Times Op-Ed:* Farris, Grace. "Fighting Coronavirus Means I Haven't Seen My Kids for a Month." *The New York Times,* 15 Apr. 2020, www.nytimes.com/2020/04/15/parenting/coronavirus-doctor-family.html. Dr. Farris left the Mount Sinai Health System in the summer of 2020 for The University of Texas at Austin's Dell Medical School.

125 *Joanne Hojsak:* from the Mount Sinai Archives project, COVID Memories.

125 *Matthew Bai:* "From the Frontlines: Dr. Matthew Bai's Story." YouTube, Mount Sinai Health System, 3 Apr. 2020, www.youtube.com/watch?v=c5bS4lPnJdg.

126 *April 4 video diary:* "From the Frontlines: Dr. Sanam Ahmed's Story." YouTube, Mount Sinai Health System, 7 Apr. 2020, www.youtube.com/watch?v=rcGxnNBLBWA.

127 *Umesh Gidwani captured his thoughts:* "Coronavirus Outbreak: New York Doctor Shows Day in Life at Hospital During COVID-19 Crisis." YouTube, Global News, 3 Apr. 2020, www.youtube.com/watch?v=pCslPGBJ4jI.

CHAPTER 8

132 *in Academic Medicine:* Bahethi, Rohini R., et al. "The COVID-19 Student Workforce at the Icahn School of Medicine at Mount Sinai: A Model for Rapid Response in Emergency Preparedness." *Academic Medicine,* vol. 96, no. 6, June 2021, pp. 859–863, doi:10.1097/acm.0000000000003863. (published online December 2020)

134 *said David Thomas:* "New Mount Sinai Doctors among Those Making Valuable Contributions During the Pandemic." *Mount Sinai Today,* 2 July 2020, health.mountsinai.org/blog/new-mount-sinai-doctors-among those-making-valuable-contributions-during-the-pandemic/.

135 *Mount Sinai's "COVID Memories" project:* from the Mount Sinai Archives project, COVID Memories.

137 *wrote up these principles:* Muller, David, et al. "Guiding Principles for Undergraduate Medical Education in the Time of the COVID-19 Pandemic." *Medical Teacher,* vol. 43, no. 2, 3 Nov. 2020, pp. 137–141, doi:10.1080/0142159x.2020.1841892.

139 *med school applications was 18 percent:* Cranmore, Crystal. "Coronavirus Update New York City: Medical Schools Seeing Increase in Applicants Amid COVID Pandemic." *ABC7 New York,* WABC-TV, 30 Apr. 2021, abc7ny.com/health/medical-schools-seeing-increase-in-applicants-amid-coronavirus-pandemic/10553014/.

139 *3 percent:* Weiner, Stacy. "Applications to Medical School Are at an All-Time High. What Does This Mean for Applicants and Schools?" AAMC, 22 Oct. 2020, www.aamc.org/news-insights/applications-medical-school-are-all-time-high-what-does-mean-applicants-and-schools.

139 *Applications for selective colleges:* Nierenberg, Amelia. "Interest Surges in Top Colleges, While Struggling Ones Scrape for Applicants." *The New York Times,* 20 Feb. 2021, www.nytimes.com/2021/02/20/us/colleges-covid-applicants.html.

139 *says Geoffrey Young:* Weiner, "Applications to Medical School."

CHAPTER 9

142 *left noses and hands raw and bloody:* Among many skin care rituals and frontline innovations, wound care nurses at Mount Sinai Morningside came up with a dressing to protect faces beneath masks.

142 *use appropriate PPE:* Additional studies bore this out. *See:* Karlsson, Ulf, and Carl-Johan Fraenkel. "Complete Protection from COVID-19 Is Possible for Health Workers." *BMJ,* 7 July 2020, p. m2641, doi:10.1136/bmj.m2641.

143 *drive down costs: See:* Feinmann, Jane. "PPE: What Now for the Global Supply Chain?" *BMJ,* 15 May 2020, p. m1910, doi:10.1136/bmj.m1910.

143 *held fast to those resources: See:* Bradsher, Keith, and Liz Alderman. "The World Needs Masks. China Makes Them, but Has Been Hoarding Them." *The New York Times,* 13 Mar. 2020, www.nytimes.com/2020/03/13/business/masks-china-coronavirus.html.

144 *said Mr. Maceda:* The most difficult part of Carlos Maceda's job during the pandemic occurred when he mourned with his team over the COVID death of Vedat Sarayli, director of purchasing. "The hardest thing I've ever done in my career was to announce that on Zoom and hear people openly cry and not be able to console, to hug, to come together as a group and grieve together," Mr. Maceda said, praising his team for still being able to "focus on making sure that orders got placed."
    COVID did that, induced people to compartmentalize loss and grief and still carry on with the most difficult jobs of their lives.

145 *commitment never to run out:* As of September 2020, Mount Sinai Health System had at least 90 days' worth of personal protective equipment on hand, as was mandated by the state. The mandate was lowered to 60 days in 2021.

147 *placed carnations:* Bonfiglio, Briana. "Food Donations Pour in at Mount Sinai South Nassau." *Herald Community Newspapers,* 27 Mar. 2020, liherald.com/stories/food-donations-pour-in-at-mount-sinai-south-nassau,123510.

149 *shared the protocol:* "Repurposing bi-level ventilators for use with intubated

patients while minimizing risk to health care workers during insufficient supply of conventional ventilation for patients with COVID-19," https://health.mountsinai.org/wp-content/uploads/sites/14/2020/04/NIV-to-Ventilator-Modification-Protocol-v1.02-for-posting.pdf.

149 *to India:* Fiore, Kristina. "After Friend's Death, Physician Rallies Support for India's COVID Crisis." *Medical News,* MedpageToday, 5 May 2021, www.medpagetoday.com/special-reports/exclusives/92429.

150 *October 2020 issue of Anesthesiology:* Levin, Matthew A., et al. "Differential Ventilation Using Flow Control Valves as a Potential Bridge to Full Ventilatory Support during the COVID-19 Crisis." *Anesthesiology,* vol. 133, no. 4, Oct. 2020, pp. 892–904, doi:10.1097/aln.0000000000003473.

150 *Italy's overwhelmed Lombardy region:* For more, see: Rosenbaum, Lisa. "Facing COVID-19 in Italy - Ethics, Logistics, and Therapeutics on the Epidemic's Front Line." *New England Journal of Medicine,* vol. 382, no. 20, 18 Mar. 2020, pp. 1873–1875, doi:10.1056/nejmp2005492. *See also:* Mounk, Yascha. "The Extraordinary Decisions Facing Italian Doctors." *The Atlantic,* 11 Mar. 2020, www.theatlantic.com/ideas/archive/2020/03/who-gets-hospital-bed/607807/.

CHAPTER 10

156 *Esther and Joseph Klingenstein Clinical Center:* Niss, Barbara, and Arthur H. Aufses. *Teaching Tomorrow's Medicine Today: the Mount Sinai School of Medicine, 1963-2003.* New York University Press, 2005, p. 10.

157 *Hans Popper ... future setting of medicine:* Popper, Hans. "The Mount Sinai Concept." Clinical Research, XIII, № 4, 1965, pp. 500–504.

157 *remodeled bus garage:* "Mount Sinai Opens Its Medical School in Old Bus Garage." *The New York Times,* 7 Sept. 1968.

157 *the school's fiftieth anniversary:* Stark, Ellen. "50 Years of Innovation." *Mount Sinai Science & Medicine,* 2018, pp. 3–9.

158 *said Dennis Charney:* Ibid.

159 *define key characteristics:* Jacobi, Adam, et al. "Portable Chest X-Ray in Coronavirus Disease-19 (COVID-19): A Pictorial Review." *Clinical Imaging,* vol. 64, Aug. 2020, pp. 35–42, doi:10.1016/j.clinimag.2020.04.001. (published online 8 Apr. 2020)

159 *augmented by artificial intelligence:* Mei, Xueyan, et al. "Artificial Intelligence–Enabled Rapid Diagnosis of Patients with COVID-19." *Nature Medicine,* vol. 26, no. 8, 19 May 2020, pp. 1224–1228, doi:10.1038/s41591-020-0931-3.

159 *enrolled the health system:* See also: "Behind the Scenes With Judith Aberg, MD, a Leader in Mount Sinai's COVID-19 Response." *Mount Sinai Today,* 18 Nov. 2020, health.mountsinai.org/blog/behind-the-scenes-with-judith-aberg-md-a-leader-in-mount-sinais-covid-19-response/.

160 *COVID-19 infection during pregnancy:* "Thousands of Mothers Take Part in Mount Sinai Study of COVID-19 and Pregnancy." *Mount Sinai Today,* 11 May 2021, health.mountsinai.org/blog/thousands-of-mothers-take-part-in-mount-sinai-study-of-covid-19-and-pregnancy/.

160 *hydroxychloroquine:* "We did the same as everybody else, jumped on the

bandwagon that hydroxychloroquine may be a benefit based on data that was coming initially from China and Europe," said infectious diseases head Judith Aberg. "But I will tell you that we started noting harm even before the EUA was withdrawn." Mount Sinai then stopped the treatment. "Because our health system is so large," said Dr. Aberg, "we were able to pick up on things that may be beneficial or may be harmful even before the trial results were coming out."

161 *more than $70 million:* Reflecting a remarkable degree of urgency and of community support, the $70 million that Mount Sinai raised in the first *six months* of the pandemic was more than it had ever raised in an entire fiscal year, in the health system's history.

164 *harm's way," said Dr. Krammer:* "Prof. Florian Krammer: Life in a Virus Lab during the COVID-19 Pandemic." TIPS (The Infection Prevention Strategy), 20 July 2020, deepdive.tips/index.php/2020/07/20/prof-florian-krammer-life-in-a-virus-lab-during-the-covid-19-pandemic/.

164 *Dr. Merad wrote in Nature Medicine:* Merad, Miriam. "Reflections from a Mother Scientist." *Nature Medicine,* vol. 26, no. 9, 24 Aug. 2020, pp. 1316–1316, doi:10.1038/s41591-020-1052-8.

CHAPTER 11

167 *Facebook Live presentation:* "COVID-19 Research: On the Front Lines." Facebook, U.S. Embassy Paris, 5 May 2000, www.facebook.com/watch/live/?v=335675584077669&ref=watch_permalink.
Dr. tenOever left Mount Sinai for NYU Langone in 2021.

167 *As Michiko Kakutani wrote:* Kakutani, Michiko. "The 2010s Were the End of Normal." *The New York Times,* 27 Dec. 2019, www.nytimes.com/interactive/2019/12/27/opinion/sunday/2010s-america-trump.html?action=click&module=RelatedLinks&pgtype=Article.

167 *released the genomic sequence:* "Severe Acute Respiratory Syndrome CORONAVIRUS 2 Isolate WUHAN-HU-1, CO - Nucleotide - NCBI." *National Center for Biotechnology Information,* U.S. National Library of Medicine, www.ncbi.nlm.nih.gov/nuccore/MN908947.

168 *according to the CDC:* "SARS (10 Years After)." Centers for Disease Control and Prevention, 3 Mar. 2016, www.cdc.gov/dotw/sars/index.html.

168 *who was a boy in China:* "Prof. Florian Krammer: Life in a Virus Lab," TIPS.

168 *2003 SARS-CoV-1 numbers:* "SARS (10 Years After)." Centers for Disease Control and Prevention, 3 Mar. 2016, www.cdc.gov/dotw/sars/index.html.

168 *New York Times Op-Ed:* Kilbourne, Edwin D. "Flu to the Starboard! Man the Harpoons! Fill 'Em With Vaccine! Get the Captain! Hurry!" *The New York Times,* 13 Feb. 1976, nyti.ms/1kpkhO8.

169 *using sequences:* "Peter Palese: 'Pandemic Diseases.'" YouTube, Howard Hughes Medical Institute, 13 May 2021, www.youtube.com/watch?v=AYEYk5FsTwU.

169 *New York Times Op-Ed:* Kilbourne.

170 *sickened more than 60 million:* "2009 H1N1 Pandemic." Centers for Disease Control and Prevention, 11 June 2019, www.cdc.gov/flu/pandemic-resources/2009-h1n1-pandemic.html#:~:text=From%20April%2012%2C%202009%20to,the%20(H1N1)pdm09%20virus.

170 *people over sixty-five:* Manicassamy, Balaji, et al. "Protection of Mice against Lethal Challenge with 2009 H1N1 Influenza a Virus by 1918-Like and Classical Swine H1N1 Based Vaccines." *PLoS Pathogens,* vol. 6, no. 1, 29 Jan. 2010, doi:10.1371/journal.ppat.1000745.

170 *Centers of Excellence:* "Centers of Excellence for Influenza Research and Response (CEIRR)." National Institute of Allergy and Infectious Diseases, U.S. Department of Health and Human Services, www.niaid.nih.gov/research/centers-excellence-influenza-research-response.

In May 2021, the Icahn School was awarded its third seven-year contract for the Center by the NIH's National Institute of Allergy and Infectious Diseases (NIAID), a grant valued at $42 million. Over its next seven years, the influenza-focused Center of Excellence planned to expand to include research into treatments and prevention of SARS-CoV-2.

172 *Benjamin tenOever described:* Blanco-Melo, Daniel, et al. "Imbalanced Host Response to SARS-CoV-2 Drives Development of COVID-19." *Cell,* vol. 181, no. 5, 15 May 2020, doi:10.1016/j.cell.2020.04.026.

172 *This shed light:* The discovery helped prompt colleagues in the Precision Immunology Institute to write a clinical trial to test an existing recombinant interferon treatment in COVID patients. The trial was written in a record seventy-two hours and opened within a month and a half, as opposed to, more typically, a year and a half, said principal investigator Thomas Marron, who is a cancer immunologist. In the end, it did not get off the ground, as its launch in May coincided with a precipitous drop in COVID patients, and doctors were unable to enroll enough patients at Mount Sinai.

172 *Microbiologist Benhur Lee:* "Mount Sinai Develops 'Pseudo Virus' to Assess the Effectiveness of Antibodies." *Mount Sinai Today,* 30 Apr. 2020, health.mountsinai.org/blog/mount-sinai-develops-pseudo-virus-to-assess-the-effectiveness-of-antibodies/.

173 *published in Science:* White, Kris M., et al. "Plitidepsin Has Potent Preclinical Efficacy Against SARS-CoV-2 by Targeting the Host Protein EEF1A." *Science,* vol. 371, no. 6532, 26 Feb. 2021, pp. 926–931, doi:10.1126/science.abf4058.

173 *emerged from the pharmaceutical industry:* These included mRNA vaccines from Pfizer and Moderna, as well as adenovirus-vector vaccines from Johnson & Johnson and AstraZeneca.

173 *universal flu vaccine:* In preparing to teach his class on emerging viruses again in 2021, Dr. Krammer revisited notes from the last time he taught the class, in 2019. He found what he called "this pre-pandemic gem." An assignment asked students to develop a case for study and presentation, and one of the case options was:
> *1) We have heard of SARS CoV and MERS CoV which rarely cause disease in humans. Which other coronaviruses circulate in humans? What type of disease do they cause? When/how were they discovered?*
> *2) How would you design a vaccine that protects against all coronavirus infections?*
Source: Florian Krammer's twitter account, @florian_krammer, 25 Apr. 2021.

177 *seminal paper:* Amanat, Fatima, et al. "A Serological Assay to Detect SARS-CoV-2 Seroconversion in Humans." *Nature Medicine,* vol. 26, no. 7, July 2020, pp. 1033–1036, doi:10.1038/s41591-020-0913-5. (preprinted online 16 April)

177 *This Week in Virology:* "TWiV 638: Do, There Is No Try: This Week in Virology."

This Week in Virology | A Podcast about Viruses - the Kind That Make You Sick, 5 Aug. 2020, www.microbe.tv/twiv/twiv-638/.

178 *as a qualitative test:* "Mount Sinai's Blood Test to Detect Antibodies to COVID-19 Receives Emergency Use Authorization from U.S. Food and Drug Administration." Mount Sinai Health System, 15 Apr. 2020, www.mountsinai.org/about/newsroom/2020/mount-sinais-blood-test-to-detect-antibodies-to-covid19-receives-emergency-use-authorization-from-us-food-and-drug-administration-pr.

178 *as a quantitative test:* "New York State Department of Health Grants Emergency Use Authorization to Mount Sinai for Quantitative COVID-19 Antibody Test." Mount Sinai Health System, 17 Sept. 2020, www.mountsinai.org/about/newsroom/2020/new-york-state-department-of-health-grants-emergency-use-authorization-to-mount-sinai-for-quantitative-covid19-antibody-test-pr.

178 *more than 145,000 and more than 4.3 million:* COVID-19 Map. Johns Hopkins.

179 *Anderson Cooper and CNN:* "CNN Interview: Florian Krammer, PhD, Discusses Antibodies, Immunity, and COVID-19." Physician's Channel - Mount Sinai New York, 29 Apr. 2020, physicians.mountsinai.org/videos/cnn-interview-florian-krammer-phd-discusses-antibodies-immunity-and-covid-19.

179 *National Public Radio:* Harris, Richard. "Studies Suggest Immunity to the Coronavirus Is Likely to Be Short Term." NPR, 22 July 2020, www.npr.org/2020/07/22/894343521/studies-suggest-immunity-to-the-coronavirus-is-likely-to-be-short-term.

179 *high school students:* Wu, Katherine J. "Amid One Pandemic, Students Train for the Next." *The New York Times,* 21 Jan. 2021, www.nytimes.com/2021/01/21/health/coronavirus-education-high-school.html.

179 *in the Lancet Microbe:* Wajnberg, Ania, et al. "Humoral Response and PCR Positivity in Patients With COVID-19 in the New York City Region, USA: An Observational Study." The Lancet Microbe, vol. 1, no. 7, 25 Sept. 2020, doi:10.1016/s2666-5247(20)30120-8. (preprinted online July)

179 *published in Science in December:* Wajnberg, Ania, et al. "Robust Neutralizing Antibodies to SARS-CoV-2 Infection Persist for Months." *Science,* 4 Dec. 2020, www.ncbi.nlm.nih.gov/pmc/articles/PMC7810037/. (preprinted online October)

182 *too large to control:* "TWiV 638".

184 *later published in Science:* Gonzalez-Reiche, Ana S., et al. "Introductions and Early Spread of SARS-CoV-2 in the New York City Area." *Science,* vol. 369, no. 6501, 17 July 2020, pp. 297–301, doi:10.1126/science.abc1917. (preprinted online April)

184 *bolstered by a subsequent study:* Stadlbauer, Daniel, et al. "Repeated Cross-Sectional Sero-Monitoring of SARS-CoV-2 in New York City." *Nature,* vol. 590, no. 7844, 3 Nov. 2020, pp. 146–150, doi:10.1038/s41586-020-2912-6.

CHAPTER 12

190 *she told CBS's 60 Minutes:* "Puzzling, Often Debilitating After-Effects Plaguing COVID-19 'Long-Haulers.'" CBS News (60 Minutes), 20 Nov. 2020, www.cbsnews.com/news/covid-long-haulers-60-minutes-2020-11-22/?ftag=CNM-00-10aab5j&linkId=105167416&fbclid=IwAR2nQwrV9st7elRgfumuoQy9mXtX-TKBMXn3yDdsiOIr1GtkAD9RgnvhsENs.

191 *published in Modern Pathology:* Bryce, Clare, et al. "Pathophysiology of SARS-CoV-2."

193 *neurological sequelae beginning to emerge:* ibid.

197 *published in Nature Medicine:* Del Valle.

198 *RECOVERY trial:* RECOVERY Collaborative Group. "Tocilizumab in Patients Admitted to Hospital with COVID-19 (RECOVERY): a Randomised, Controlled, Open-Label, Platform Trial." *The Lancet,* 1 May 2021, www.thelancet.com/journals/lancet/article/PIIS0140-6736(21)00676-0/fulltext.

200 *high-impact mobilization:* Charney, Alexander W., et al. "Sampling the Host Response to SARS-CoV-2 in Hospitals under Siege." *Nature Medicine,* vol. 26, no. 8, 27 July 2020, pp. 1157–1158, doi:10.1038/s41591-020-1004-3.

201 *set of matched controls:* In the fog-of-war atmosphere, drawing samples from controls almost fell through the cracks, until Noam Beckmann, the genetic and genomic scientist leading the biobank's data generation, remembered to write it into the specs. "We were thinking so much about collecting data from individuals with COVID-19 that everyone forgot that we needed controls. And without controls, you can't ask any questions," he said, noting that matched controls were hard to come by during the peak, because there were so few non-COVID patients coming to the hospitals. "I believe that's one of my biggest contributions scientifically to this endeavor."

202 *largely empty Hess Building:* For Alex Charney, the bustling biobank team's spread across the fifth and sixth floors of an otherwise shuttered research nerve center was both hopeful and haunting. "The hospitals were overwhelmed, but on the research side—which is a big part of Mount Sinai—it was like a ghost town," said Dr. Charney. "It was like you were the only person left on Earth."

CHAPTER 13

210 *only outside models available:* The two U.S. models widely used at the time to forecast COVID patient census were the University of Pennsylvania's CHIME (COVID-19 Hospital Impact Model for Epidemics) model and the University of Washington's IHME (Institute of Health Metrics and Evaluation) model.

211 *2,000 patients on April 10:* Different sources recorded patient census and other statistics differently. The daily forecast, and many Mount Sinai clinicians and hospital leaders, reported the 2,000 figure. This book, unless otherwise noted (e.g., here), uses retrospective figures from the electronic medical record, which had the peak at April 7, with 1,641 COVID-positive patients.

213 *acute kidney injury:* Chan, Lili, et al. "AKI in Hospitalized Patients With COVID-19." *Journal of the American Society of Nephrology,* vol. 32, no. 1, Jan. 2021, pp. 151–160, doi:10.1681/asn.2020050615.

213 *suffered from myocardial injury:* Lala, Anuradha, et al. "Prevalence and Impact of Myocardial Injury in Patients Hospitalized with COVID-19 Infection." *Journal of the American College of Cardiology,* vol. 76, no. 5, Aug. 2020, pp. 533–546.

213 *COVID-19," said Dr. Hirten:* "Mount Sinai Researchers Use Apple Watch to Predict COVID-19." *Mount Sinai Today,* 4 Dec. 2020, health.mountsinai.org/blog/mount-sinai-researchers-use-apple-watch-to-predict-covid-19/.

214 *study published in September 2021:* Hirten, Robert P, et al. "Factors Associated with Longitudinal Psychological and Physiological Stress in Health Care Workers during the COVID-19 Pandemic: Observational Study Using Apple Watch Data." *Journal of Medical Internet Research,* vol. 23, no. 9, 13 Sept. 2021, doi:10.2196/31295. *See also:* "Mount Sinai Researchers Use Wearable Devices to Identify Psychological Effects of Pandemic." *Mount Sinai Health System,* Mount Sinai Health System, 13 Sept. 2021, www.mountsinai.org/about/newsroom/2021/mount-sinai-researchers-use-wearable-devices-to-identify-psychological-effects-of-pandemic.

214 *mental health supports they need:* In spring 2021, Drs. Fayad and Hirten launched a third element of the Warrior Watch—the Warrior Shield, which, through the mobile app, seeks to build resilience using biofeedback.

215 *50 percent higher chance:* The study was published in JACC in October 2020 and built off a smaller study published online in May 2020, just weeks after the anticoagulation protocol went into effect at Mount Sinai. *See:* Nadkarni, Girish N., et al. "Anticoagulation, Bleeding, Mortality, and Pathology in Hospitalized Patients With COVID-19." *Journal of the American College of Cardiology,* vol. 76, no. 16, Oct. 2020, pp. 1815–1826.

216 *According to the CDC:* "Risk for COVID-19 Infection, Hospitalization, and Death by Race/Ethnicity." Centers for Disease Control and Prevention, www.cdc.gov/coronavirus/2019-ncov/covid-data/investigations-discovery/hospitalization-death-by-race-ethnicity.html.

222 *Ms. Finley told the Road to Resilience podcast:* "Workshopping Resilience." Mount Sinai Health System, Road to Resilience Podcast, 6 Nov. 2020, www.mountsinai.org/about/newsroom/podcasts/road-resilience/workshopping-resilience.

222 *said about the evidence-based workshops:* "Resilience: An Introduction." YouTube, Icahn School of Medicine, 11 Nov. 2020, www.youtube.com/watch?v=I1M1F04HNvs.

223 *one of ten resilience factors:* Southwick, Steven M., and Dennis S. Charney. *Resilience: The Science of Mastering Life's Greatest Challenges.* Cambridge University Press, 2014.

225 *in the Journal of the American Medical Association:* Shanafelt, Tait, et al. "Understanding and Addressing Sources of Anxiety among Health Care Professionals during the COVID-19 Pandemic." *JAMA,* vol. 323, no. 21, 7 Apr. 2020, pp. 2133–2134, doi:10.1001/jama.2020.5893.

226 *study of more than 4,000 World Trade Center responders:* Chen, Connie, et al. "The Burden of Subthreshold Posttraumatic Stress Disorder in World Trade Center Responders in the Second Decade after 9/11." *The Journal of Clinical Psychiatry,* vol. 81, no. 1, 21 Jan. 2020, doi:10.4088/jcp.19m12881.

CHAPTER 14

231 *retrospective observational study:* Tabacof, Laura, et al. "Post-Acute COVID-19 Syndrome Negatively Impacts Health and Wellbeing Despite Less Severe Acute Infection." MedRxiv, 6 Nov. 2020, doi:10.1101/2020.11.04.20226126.

231 *Center for Post-COVID Care launched in May 2020:* Fifteen months after

opening, as of August 2021, Mount Sinai's Center for Post-COVID Care had treated some 3,000 patients.

237 *said the CDC guidelines:* "Key Points." Centers for Disease Control and Prevention, www.cdc.gov/coronavirus/2019-ncov/hcp/clinical-care/post-covid-index.html.
  The CDC consulted with, among others, patient advocacy groups that included Survivor Corps, which had led Caitlin Barber to Mount Sinai. *See also:* Cirruzzo, Chelsea. "The CDC Has New Guidance on Treating Long COVID." *U.S. News & World Report,* 15 June 2021, www.usnews.com/news/healthiest-communities/articles/2021-06-15/cdc-releases-guidance-to-providers-on-treating-long-covid.

CHAPTER 15

239 *said David Reich:* "Lessons from the Epicenter: What We Have Learned about COVID-19." *Mount Sinai Today,* 12 June 2020, health.mountsinai.org/blog/lessons-from-the-epicenter-what-we-have-learned-about-covid-19/.

242 *COVID-19 Clinical Rounds:* From March 2020 to August 2021, the program reached more than 51,000 participants. For more on the COVID-19 Clinical Rounds Initiative, see: Hunt, Richard C., et al. "Virtual Peer-to-Peer Learning to Enhance and Accelerate the Health System Response to COVID-19: The HHS ASPR Project ECHO COVID-19 Clinical Rounds Initiative," *Annals of Emergency Medicine,* vol. 78, no. 2, Aug. 2021, pp. 223–228, doi:10.1016/j.annemergmed.2021.03.035.

242 *After-action reports:* National Dialogue for Healthcare Innovation; Duke Margolis Center for Health Policy. *National Dialogue for Healthcare Innovation: Framework for Private-Public Collaboration on Disaster Preparedness and Response,* Feb. 2021.

245 *9/11 Commission cited:* Kean, Thomas H., and Lee H. Hamilton. *The 9/11 Commission Report: Final Report of the National Commission on Terrorist Attacks upon the United States,* Norton, 2004, pp. 339-344. The report goes on to concede, "Imagination is not a gift usually associated with bureaucracies."

246 *Op-Ed in The Hill:* Davis, Kenneth L. and Brendan Carr, opinion contributors. "The Next Pandemic Is Coming. Will We Be Prepared?" *The Hill,* 23 Mar. 2021, thehill.com/opinion/healthcare/544592-the-next-pandemic-is-coming-will-we-be-prepared.

247 *more than ten states:* Stone, Will. "A COVID Surge Is Overwhelming U.S. Hospitals, Raising Fears of Rationed Care." *NPR,* 5 Sept. 2021, www.npr.org/sections/health-shots/2021/09/05/1034210487/covid-surge-overwhelming-hospitals-raising-fears-rationed-care.

247 *ICUs more than 95 percent full:* Smart, Charlie. "COVID Hospitalization Crisis Reaches Fever Pitch in Southern I.C.U.s." *The New York Times,* 14 Sept. 2021, www.nytimes.com/interactive/2021/09/14/us/covid-hospital-icu-south.html.

247 *parking garages across the South:* Maan, Anurag, and Julia Harte. "Mississippi Hospital Puts Beds in Parking Garage to Cope with COVID-19 Surge." *Reuters,* 14 Aug. 2021, www.reuters.com/world/us/mississippi-hospital-puts-beds-parking-garage-cope-with-covid-19-surge-2021-08-13/.

248 *The Lens podcast:* "Podcast, the Lens, COVID-19 Episode #2 - Learnings from a New York City Hospital - Part 1." *Catalysis,* createvalue.org/articles_and_news/podcast-lens-covid-19-episode-2-learnings-new-york-city-hospital-part-1/.

248 *Dr. Boal pointed out:* Radio Advisory.

250 *Findings in a Lancet:* Prasad, Kriti, et al. "Prevalence and Correlates of Stress and Burnout among U.S. Healthcare Workers During the COVID-19 Pandemic: A National Cross-Sectional Survey Study." *EClinicalMedicine,* vol. 35, 16 May 2021, p. 100879, doi:10.1016/j.eclinm.2021.100879.

251 *1 in 500 Americans:* Keating, Dan, et al. "The Pandemic Marks Another Grim Milestone: 1 in 500 Americans Have Died of COVID-19." *The Washington Post,* 15 Sept. 2021, www.washingtonpost.com/health/interactive/2021/1-in-500-covid-deaths/.